D0469603

"*Live Long, Die Short* is the Rosetta Stone o. written by Dr. Roger Landry, this book translates the most up-to-date science related to human wellness and vitality into an engaging guide to a better life. I especially appreciated Dr. Landry's fluid, reassuring prose. He has a bright future as a writer."

— **William Thomas, MD, founder of the Eden Alternative; author of**
What Are Old People For: How Elders Will Save the World

"The philosopher Camus once said something like this: 'In the depth of winter, I finally learned that within me there lay an invincible summer.' Roger Landry's book is the invincible summer human operator's manual. It blows up long-standing aging stereotypes and self-fulfilling prophecies and replaces them with evidenced-based attitudes and behaviors that can transform the aging experience for each of us, and for those whose lives we touch every day. None of us wants to age. Yet, our attitudes, our lifestyle, and our management of inevitable health conditions built into our gene pool or caused by chance are factors we can either accept, manage, or change our outlook about so as to maximize the fulfillment of life as we age. A must-read—even more: a must-reference. The Dr. Spock book for aging! Keep it on the shelf and dog-ear parts that you will refer back to often. Roger's book is well done, honest, and hopeful."

— **Larry Minnix, president and CEO of LeadingAge**

"In *Live Long, Die Short*, Dr. Roger Landry presents a wealth of practical and scientifically sound recommendations on what it takes to age successfully. This book not only provides readers with implementable, life-altering strategies but also educates them about the human potential that exists in later life. It will change your expectations of aging. *Live Long, Die Short* is a must-read for everyone who cares about living well at any age."

— **Colin Milner, CEO of the International Council on Active Aging**

"Dr Landry's message is that both society and the individual can do much more to ensure we live our best lives as we age. He is a pioneer in his field, and his holistic approach in *Live Long, Die Short* will resonate across generations."

— **James Taylor, president, Division Southeast,**
Sodexo Healthcare Services

"Ten thousand Baby Boomers turn sixty-five each day, all marching to a destination, in fact to many different destinations. Now, they've got a road map to chart their journey into later life. Dr. Landry is the physician we've been waiting for. Now he's written us all a prescription that will help us reach our goal of successful aging."
—**Harry R. Moody, PhD, retired vice president at AARP, author**

"*Live Long, Die Short* provides us with a road map to truly maximize not only quantity but also quality of life. Dr. Landry has clearly illuminated the path and taught us that each and every one of us in the driver's seat and in control of how we age."
—**Robert Winningham, PhD, author of *Train Your Brain: How to Maximize Memory Ability in Older Adulthood*; psychology professor and chair of the Psychology Division at Western Oregon University**

"At last, some practical guidance on aging better. Dr. Landry's empathetic yet motivating message is a breath of fresh air. Authentic health! This concept is so simple and rational, yet a breakthrough in our understanding of what makes us healthy. *Live Long, Die Short* is a must-read for all who struggle to age in a better way."
—**Charles H. Roadman II, MD, Air Force Surgeon General, retired; former CEO and president of Assisted Living Concepts Inc.**

Age well ... Regularly

LIVE LONG, DIE SHORT

A Guide *to* Authentic Health
and Successful Aging

ROGER LANDRY, MD, MPH

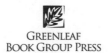

GREENLEAF
BOOK GROUP PRESS

This book is intended as a reference volume only, not as a medical manual. The information given here is designed to help you make informed decisions about your health. It is not intended as a substitute for any treatment that may have been prescribed by your doctor. If you suspect that you have a medical problem, you should seek competent medical help. You should not begin a new health regimen without first consulting a medical professional.

Published by Greenleaf Book Group Press
Austin, Texas
www.gbgpress.com

Distributed by Greenleaf Book Group LLC

For ordering information or special discounts for bulk purchases, please contact Greenleaf Book Group LLC at PO Box 91869, Austin, TX 78709, 512.891.6100.

Design, Cover Design, and composition by Greenleaf Book Group LLC
Cover illustration (tree): ©iStockphoto.com/paci77

Cataloging-in-Publication data
Landry, Roger, 1946-
　Live long, die short : a guide to authentic health and successful aging/Roger Landry.—1st ed.
　　p. : ill. ; cm.
　Includes bibliographical references.
　Issued also as an ebook.
　ISBN: 978-1-62634-073-2 (hardcover)
　ISBN: 978-1-62634-039-8 (pbk.)
　1. Older people—Health and hygiene. 2. Aging. I. Title.

RA777.6 .L36 2014
613/.0438　　　　　　　　　　　　　　　　　　　2013947767

Part of the Tree Neutral® program, which offsets the number of trees consumed in the production and printing of this book by taking proactive steps, such as planting trees in direct proportion to the number of trees used: www.treeneutral.com

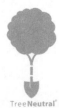

TreeNeutral®

Printed in the United States of America on acid-free paper

17 18 19 20 21 10 9 8 7 6 5 4

First Edition

FOR MOM AND DAD

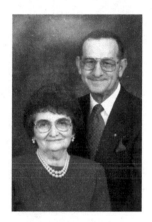

*Lucky parents who have fine children usually have
lucky children who have fine parents.*

—JAMES A. BREWER

ACKNOWLEDGMENTS

I never could have written this book without help: inspiration from the magnificent Masterpiece Living Team for what they have achieved in changing aging in this country; support and opportunity from my brother, Larry, a visionary who continues to surprise me; the prodding of my good friend George Devins; the fabulous Greenleaf staff; encouragement from the hundreds of older adults who graciously urged me to write down the words I shared with them in their lecture halls, dining areas, and living rooms over the last fifteen years, and many of whom in turn shared their inspiring life stories with me; the understanding of those most prominent in my world: Paula, my wife and lifelong companion, my inspiring adult children, Jen and Jeff, and supportive close friends—all of whom allowed me to be periodically absent from my life during the last year in order to bring an idea to reality; and most of all, Jackson, Dylan, Hunter, and Abigail, my grandchildren, who unknowingly kept me at the computer with a hope of making their world better than mine.

CONTENTS

FOREWORD

This is a remarkable book—remarkable for its candor, its range, and, most important, for the scientific validity of its information about how to age successfully.

Candor: This book is not an autobiography, but in the course of explaining his current work and his dedication to a health-promoting lifestyle, Dr. Landry is candid about his own life and his career of twenty-three years in the US Air Force. He is explicit about the disappointing discovery, shortly after his retirement from the Air Force, that his central emphasis as a physician—preventing disease and deterioration—was considered, at least by some medical providers, as an unprofitable alternative to dramatic and expensive repairs of damage already done. Finally, he is candid about his enthusiasm for the accumulating evidence that a combination of diet, exercise, supportive social relations, and productive activity can really bring people closer to a better aging experience.

Range: Roger Landry's main purpose in writing this book is to enable people to live long and successfully. In an uncertain world, nothing can guarantee this outcome for each individual, but the accumulating experience of doctors and medical researchers can teach us a great deal about how to improve the odds in our favor. Dr. Landry's knowledge about successful aging has the depth and practicality that comes from the combination of research and direct doctor-patient experience. The book also includes a kind of autobiographical subtext that adds to both a reader's interest and confidence in its advice.

That story line takes us from Landry's graduation from Tufts medical school to his twenty-three years in the Air Force, from which he retired as Chief Flight Surgeon with a rank of colonel. That long career was followed by a shorter interval in the private healthcare industry, and now a third career as a key player in the development and demonstration of a life-changing pattern of successful aging, and as president of an organization that aims to make that pattern increasingly visible and effective in retirement communities. Nor is this the end of the story. Roger Landry is acutely aware of the fact that successful aging in upscale retirement communities, encouraging and crucial as it is, leaves important questions still to be answered: whether and how those opportunities and that lifestyle can be made available to the larger population of low-income, affordable-care residents, and how it can be extended to the far larger population of older men and women who choose—insist—on remaining in their homes, homes chosen without regard to the limitations of old age but filled with the memories and the physical reminders of earlier years and family life.

Scientific validity: Potential readers of this book should not assume that its colloquial title and its intimate, conversational style involve a casual attitude toward scientific data. The hyphenated adjective **evidence-based** is far more prevalent than the serious demand for evidence and the recognition of its presence or absence. Roger Landry is tough-minded about these issues, and his book benefits from that fact. Masterpiece Living, the initiative that he describes in the initial and final sections of his book, came out of research: ten years of surveys and experiments supported by the MacArthur Foundation and the National Institutes of Health. The Masterpiece Living organization continues to add to that knowledge base, by evaluation of its own efforts at application.

I conclude this brief foreword with a personal note. In my world of academic research, statements about possible conflicts of interest are now required, so here is mine: I have been involved in the development of Masterpiece Living. However, my participation is unpaid, so while my judgment may be biased in its favor, it is not by reimbursement.

Finally, I write this as I am about to celebrate my ninety-fifth birthday. I try to follow the combination of diet, exercise, social relations, and productive activity that is advocated in this book. As to whether I have lived my whole life this way, I reply as a terse New Englander did to a similar question: "Not yet!"

Read this book. You will certainly enjoy it. You will almost certainly learn from it. And most important, it may bring you closer to attaining the ideal of its title: live long, die short.

—Robert L. Kahn, PhD
Ann Arbor, Michigan

WHY THIS BOOK?

People write books for many reasons. For me, it wasn't an easy decision. With so many fine books on aging by experienced and gifted authors, I wondered what I might add to the accumulating mountain of knowledge on the topic. So I procrastinated. That, as it turned out, was a good thing. It allowed, my friend Bill Crawford tells me, my unique voice to develop further. It allowed the varied elements of my experience—preventive medicine, public health, social research on aging, an avid interest in cultural and biological anthropology, and forty years of attempting to keep people healthy and performing at their best—to simmer, stew, and blend until the end result was indeed unique. It was that uniqueness that cried out for expression. I knew then I had to write this book. Without that procrastination, that ripening of my accumulated experience, I would never have undertaken this journey, or, having begun it prematurely, I would have fallen victim to the lonely and emotionally challenging process of bringing a book to life, and never finished.

And isn't that a metaphor of sorts? In a book about aging, about what eons of human experience have taught us about being healthy and fulfilled, about the potential pitfalls of pursuing untested or immature concepts about health and aging, isn't it fitting that its writing be a long and thoughtful journey? And isn't it also fitting that this author went through periods of uncertainty, changing views, and development to reach a broader vision? Indeed, like all of us, the idea needed time to mature.

Since we're going to travel this road together, allow me to introduce myself—in single words. Humanist, husband, father, grandfather, brother, animal lover, naturalist, speaker, writer, biker, horseman, physician, kayaker, traveler, meditator, vegetarian, beachcomber, hiker, Europhile, music lover, pro-military, antiwar, procrastinator, pack rat, cross-country skier, secular, health conscious, romantic, movie lover . . . OK, you get it. The trait I hold most dear, however, is humanist.

One of the more pressing questions facing humanity today is simply stated: How do we achieve and maintain health as we age? I wrote *Live Long, Die Short* to offer you a harbor in a storm. We are bombarded with the latest research report, with the newest diet, the next miracle fitness machine, all of which claim to help us stay healthy, live longer, to even fight aging (good luck with that!). It's not that many of these new discoveries don't have value, but the barrage of claims, many contradictory, many just plain erroneous, have us chasing our tails as we seek to age in a better way. And so. *Live Long, Die Short* is meant to be a practical guide. It answers questions such as

- What can I do to stay independent?
- How can I live life to the fullest for as long as possible?
- How do I lower the likelihood that I'll get Alzheimer's disease?
- How can I minimize the effect of diseases and conditions on my life and on my family?
- What are my risks for decline and what should I do to lower those risks?
- Can I really change my lifestyle?
- How will the aging of America affect my life and that of my family?

Be reassured that you are not alone if you are struggling with these questions. My goal is to offer you answers and, more importantly, to provide you basic knowledge and tools with which to evaluate the endless assault of new and often sensational claims you face every day in your quest for better health. Rather than give you the proverbial fish, I wish to teach you to fish. I offer you a gold standard to assess any health claims, a standard based on what we humans require to maintain health and to age well, a set of necessities I call *authentic needs*. "Authentic" because they are solidly based on who we are as humans. "Authentic" because these needs are firmly established over the eons of time man has walked the earth and because they are durable despite the dramatic changes in how humans live today. An appreciation and understanding of these authentic needs will act as true north as you maneuver through the stormy seas of new "discoveries," of quick-fix solutions to complex issues of aging, of "anti-aging" claims. Understanding these needs will help you realize that aging is fundamentally a gift, a natural and wonder-filled process, which despite its highs and lows can lead to an outcome we all want and can achieve: authentic health and successful aging.

Another goal of this book is to present a challenge to each one of you, to your organizations, and to our towns, cities, and society—a challenge to incorporate what we have learned about aging into our opinions, practices, and very way of living, so that all can reach their full potential at any age. The aging of our population leaves us a choice: grow or decline. Either we provide environments and public policy that allow older adults to grow or our very societies will decline with them. *Live Long, Die Short* is a call to action, for just as Albert Einstein admonished—"Those who have the privilege to know, have the duty to act"—we all, knowing what is possible, cannot accept the status quo of aging as decline. Whether in our private lives or in the public policy we accept, we must speak out for a more enlightened view.

Live Long, Die Short is also the story of my journey with Masterpiece Living, an exciting organization that has accelerated a movement to change how we age. This book is the encapsulation of what my associates at Masterpiece Living and I have learned over the last fourteen years from older adults striving to age in a better way, from researchers, and from the outcomes and observations of thousands of aging men and women. What is particularly unique about this book, however, is that we have resisted the common impulse to merely report findings and recommend that the reader change accordingly. Rather, we have evaluated our newly acquired knowledge in context. First, in the context of us as a unique species, hundreds of thousands of years in the making, formed in radically different environments than today's; second, in the context of a modern lifestyle marked by unprecedented levels of stress; and lastly, in the context of a culture with an obsession for short-term outcomes and unrealistic expectations for change, accomplishment, and success.

No matter who you are—older adult, aging boomer, college student, or anything in between—if you are reading this book, you are most likely curious, well educated, active, positive, concerned about your health, and an early adopter of new ideas. As we travel through this book together, let's have a conversation. Read, react, and perhaps we can also continue the dialogue at www.livelongdieshort.com.

This book will change your life. It will help guide you on your path to aging successfully. We have discovered that we can indeed shorten the length of our period of decline. We therefore have every reason to believe that by living a lifestyle that reduces our risks for disease and impairment, we can indeed live long also. Not like the Greek mythological unfortunate Tithonus, whose lover asked the gods to allow him to live forever without considering how he would age. Her wish was granted by Zeus, and Tithonus was doomed to live forever, getting older, declining, becoming more feeble. Rather, my goal for you is to be the very best you can be, for as long as possible; or, as the beloved Mister Spock from *Star Trek* said so well in Vulcan: *dif-tor heh smusma*, live long and prosper.

THE TIME OF OUR LIVES

Never doubt that a small group of thoughtful,
committed citizens can change the world. Indeed,
it is the only thing that ever has.

—MARGARET MEAD

I live in New England. The spectacular colors of the fall foliage are compensation for long winters, spring insects, and temperatures not so temperate. I am drawn to the brilliant reds, oranges, and yellows of autumn, and I've decided that these magnificent leaves are a metaphor for how I want to age. I want to become more colorful as I grow older; I would like to blend with others to make more beauty than I can alone; and when my time comes, I want to fall from the tree.

Yet, in the twenty-first century, the main causes of death for those of us living in developed countries have shifted from infections and accidents to chronic diseases, and I am now less likely to age according to my metaphor. Longer life expectancy, and the preeminence of heart disease, cancer, stroke, diabetes, chronic lung disease, and Alzheimer's as companions in this longer life, will statistically relegate me to an end more like a death scene from an old Western movie: long and painful (and expensive). No wonder we hear many say they have no wish to live to be a hundred. Wouldn't most of us choose quality over quantity? Wouldn't we choose to avoid what could be a decade or more of decline associated with loss: loss of function, social connection, independence, dignity, and control over our own lives?

But for most of the last century, we accepted that there was no choice. We believed either genes or luck determined how we would age. Some of us would live highly functional lives well into their ninth and even tenth decade, but these were few, and it didn't change the overall belief that aging was a crapshoot. Get through those turbulent young years and you might live long, but with a good chance of unwanted conditions continuously nipping away at the quality of your life.

Enter Jonas Salk, the medical researcher and virologist who discovered and developed the first effective vaccine against polio. As a highly influential member of the board of directors of the celebrated John D. and Catherine T. MacArthur Foundation in the early eighties, he challenged that board to study success in aging.

This approach was a breakthrough because, up to that point, researchers on aging had approached the subject only as a process of progressive decline. The focus was on the "inevitable" infirmities and how to deal with them. The Foundation, Jonas argued, should rather focus on vitality and resilience in the older adult and what it was that fostered these more successful outcomes. In 1984, the Foundation assembled the Research Network on Successful Aging, a group of sixteen experts from a variety of age-related disciplines, and began what was to be a decade-long study on aging. They wanted to provide fresh insights into aging in America. Their findings forever changed our attitudes toward aging, jolting us from the Dark Ages of our understanding of this common human experience. Their major finding? *How we age is mostly up to us*, and that conclusion rocked our stereotypes of aging to the very core.

The seed is planted

In the fall of 1991, in a taxi on its way to Chicago's O'Hare International Airport, Larry Landry's life took an unexpected turn—one that changed everything for him and perhaps for all of us. Larry, my brother, was the chief financial officer of the MacArthur Foundation, and he shared that taxi ride with Jonas Salk. Salk was filled with optimism. He had just heard the preliminary findings of the Foundation's study on aging. He told Larry that these findings had the potential to change the aging experience of all but that, to do so, the research findings would need to be applied. Larry pressed him further for clarification and Dr. Salk explained. Without application, the findings would lie fallow. Applying them meant essentially bringing them to life: having the full understanding of what successful aging is could fundamentally change the very essence or culture of a community and a society. He suggested that a senior living community would be an ideal place to begin to show what might be possible. The small size, fairly homogeneous demographic, and possibility for peer and staff reinforcement of a better lifestyle were all characteristics of an excellent social research initiative.

The seed had been planted, and although it was planted in an unlikely place and would take years to sprout, it was in safekeeping. Larry had spent his career in the financial world and had held positions as chief investment officer and chief financial officer for various not-for-profit organizations. In 1998, he founded Westport Asset Management, a company dedicated to acquiring and developing continuing-care retirement communities. That same year, Drs. Jack Rowe and Bob Kahn, lead investigators of the MacArthur Study, published *Successful Aging*, an account of the study that explained the results and debunked multiple myths about aging. Larry was ignited by the book. He knew it was time: time to answer Jonas Salk's challenge, time to make the findings of the MacArthur Study available to more people, and time to put them in a form that could change lives and societies. With Westport, Larry had access to precisely the communities Salk thought would be best to test the findings of the MacArthur Study. What he didn't have were the people to make it happen.

And so, in the latter part of 1998 and early 1999, Larry persuaded Bob Kahn and an eclectic group of experts in aging to begin exploring how to apply the research findings on aging. They would essentially be a skunkworks for the application of successful aging. Thus, the Healthy Aging Working Group came into being. The group included, in addition to Larry and Dr. Kahn, Dr. Denis Prager, former director of the MacArthur Foundation's health program and member of the Research Network on Successful Aging; Steven Blair, president and CEO of the Cooper Institute; Dr. Kathryn Hyer from the School of Aging Studies at the University of South Florida; Katie Hammond, a doctoral candidate in aging studies at the University of South Florida; and several senior-living-industry experts. Over the following months, two more members were added: Dr. Toni Antonucci, from the University of Michigan's Institute for Social Research, and Dr. Gordon Streib, noted gerontologist and sociologist from the University of Florida. The group was formidable—but it would add one more unlikely member before it would be complete.

The merging of worlds

I spent most of my adult life as an Air Force flight surgeon. My task: keep aviators healthy and performing at their best. Trained as a physician, with specialty training in aerospace medicine and occupational medicine, I experienced a military career marked by exotic travel and unique experiences. My patients, more my friends and mates, were young, vibrant, highly capable people. So how was it that I landed in the middle of a movement to change the face of aging?

On a sweltering day in September of 1981, I sat in my office next to a legend: Brigadier General Charles Yeager, the first man to fly faster than the speed of sound. "Chuck," as he was known to the rest of the world, had returned to Edwards Air Force Base in the Mojave Desert for a flight physical exam. Though retired from the Air Force and fifty-eight years old, he was still flying as a consultant to the Air Force and defense contractors. I was the chief flight surgeon at Edwards, an aviation buff, and totally in awe of the man sitting in front of me. Having completed the physical, General Yeager kicked back in his easy West Virginia way and told me stories of his more-than-illustrious career. At one point, he became quiet for a moment and then announced that he planned to break the sound barrier again on the fiftieth anniversary of the October 14, 1947, event. Most of us are reluctant to admit to huge mistakes we have made in life, but I'm owning up to this one. I responded to this announcement by telling *the* Chuck Yeager, the *Right Stuff* Chuck Yeager, that he would be seventy-four years old then. He quietly bored into me with those smiling, kindly, but now laser-sharp eyes and said, "What's your point?"

That was my first lesson in ageism. The seasoned veteran instructing the young buck, saying that age is a number and that's all. I kept in touch with Chuck Yeager, did several more physical exams on him, and derived a great deal of pleasure in hearing that he did indeed fly faster than sound on the fiftieth anniversary of the first time. And he did it again on the fifty-fifth anniversary, and on the sixtieth and, most recently, at the age of eighty-nine, on the sixty-fifth anniversary. This remarkable man helped me break some of my own barriers.

In 1995, after four years at the Air Force Surgeon General's Office in Washington, DC, as the chief flight surgeon of the Air Force and after a total of twenty-three years of service, I left the military to join a large healthcare system that wanted to develop a world-class prevention capability. Three years later, the CEO gave me feedback that provided me an "aha" moment. She told me my preventive efforts were highly successful but *were hurting revenue*. After twenty-three years in a military system that incentivized staying healthy—highly trained aviators were a key resource, as were the multimillion-dollar aircraft they flew—it was difficult to conceive of a negative side to prevention. I went home for the weekend deflated. Was there no place where there was incentive to keep people healthy other than in the military or the highly socialized countries of Europe and Canada? That Sunday evening my phone rang. It was my brother Larry calling.

He had been to Mayo Clinic recently and by chance met a former Air Force colleague of mine, Dr. Richard Hickman. In the course of their conversation, Dick Hickman talked about some of our assignments together and Larry began to think that I might be interested in helping older adults stay healthy and performing at their best, just as I had done with aircrew. He was calling to ask me to join the Healthy Aging Working Group that very weekend. I jumped at the chance.

The HAWGs begin

When Larry had asked Dr. Bob Kahn to be a part of the Healthy Aging Working Group, Bob asked, "Why are you doing this?"

Larry's answer? "Well," he said, "it's kind of self-serving."

This answer was good enough for Dr. Kahn. It went to the heart of the goal: to help *all* older adults, in fact, *all people*, to age in a better way. When Larry asked me to join, I was looking for a commitment from him. I wanted to apply the research findings of successful aging in order to change public policy. I felt, and Bob Kahn knew, that to influence the lives of a few was a noble enough goal, but to influence public policy was to have a more widespread effect that would endure over generations.

Turns out I was not alone in these big dreams. And so it was that this unlikely mix from academia, senior living, and private consulting—with collective expertise in psychology, medicine, gerontology, nursing, exercise physiology, sociology, strategic planning, business administration, and marketing—took the momentous step forward to volunteer to change our myopic views of aging . . . and to do the right thing. The members of the Healthy Aging Working Group called themselves "HAWGs" and set out cautiously, in late fall of 1999, to explore what could be done to bring research to reality, to help older adults age successfully, as defined by the MacArthur Study and the book *Successful Aging*.

It was clear from the beginning that Dr. Kahn would be the guiding force. Over eighty years old himself, he had the professional and personal experience, the academic credentials, a remarkable ability to articulate complex ideas, and a keen intelligence that was both comforting and challenging for the group. From the beginning, he insisted that, although it would be difficult to measure the effect of any interventions, since this was social—rather than clinical or experimental—research, it was absolutely necessary for us to try. He also insisted on piloting (or beta testing) whatever approach we developed before proposing it as a widespread lifestyle intervention. Larry and the group agreed. It would make all the difference.

Masterpiece Living takes shape

The MacArthur Study findings were clear: 70 percent of the physical difference and 50 percent of the intellectual difference between those who age in the usual way and those who aged more successfully was due to lifestyle—the choices we make every day. Those aging in a better way—successfully—exhibited and maintained three key behaviors or characteristics:

1. High mental and physical function
2. Low risk of disease and disease-related disability
3. Active engagement in life[1]

Rowe and Kahn, in fact, defined successful aging as the ability to maintain these three characteristics.

In a nutshell, we wanted to get people excited about living a life characterized by these traits. Our hypothesis was that if they did, it would result in a better aging experience, closer to my vision of aging like an autumn leaf. Our first task was to develop tools that would have multiple purposes: first, to allow us to assess the current lifestyle of any individual; second, to allow us to provide feedback to that individual in order to educate and motivate each to modify lifestyle as needed; and last, to provide aggregate measurement capabilities to assess the impact of our approach. We worked much like a trainer: evaluating current status, providing feedback, assisting in the development of an improvement plan, and clearly demonstrating outcomes.

So, our initial approach, now called Masterpiece Living, consisted of six steps: (1) educate older adults on the research findings and what indeed was possible, (2) give them the opportunity to take the Lifestyle Inventory (an assessment of their current lifestyle), (3) provide feedback, (4) discuss the feedback in a one-on-one or group session with a lifestyle coordinator, (5) foster empowerment with a true coaching relationship, and (6) repeat the Lifestyle Inventory in a year. After nearly two years of intermittent meetings and prolonged discussions, it was time to pilot our approach. Would it work? Would older adults be willing to take the Lifestyle Inventory? Would the feedback motivate them to make changes? Would the likelihood of their aging in a better way change over a year?

A movement

We were eager to find out the answers, and find out we did. (The details of our pilot studies, further development, and eventual dissemination of Masterpiece Living is detailed in chapter 18.) The approach worked, and worked effectively. Older adults responded to the education, information, and attention and became avid and informed consumers of how they spent their time and how they lived their lives, and as they did, their risks for impairment plummeted. We spent several more years refining our tools, and we expanded our focus more and more on developing resources to transform the *environment*, the community itself, into places where people were stimulated to age in a better way. This involved high-level and sophisticated training, for we were dealing with environments that were the products of another time, when aging was about decline and the focus was on comfort, security, and care. Now, they were becoming centers for healthy aging, destinations for older adults who wanted to continue to grow and become the very best they could be.

In 2007, we felt that Masterpiece Living was ready. We knew we were not done refining it—in fact, we would never be done—but it was time to affect more lives, time to move out to more communities. Our journey from a taxicab ride with Jonas Salk to a validated approach to successful aging may have been a long one, but we were certain it had not been wasted time. We were part of a rising movement to change aging, to make aging the rich, vital, and rewarding experience it can be.

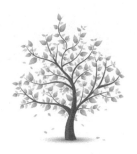

PART I

A NEW LOOK AT HEALTH, CHANGE, AND AGING

Authentic: true to one's own personality, spirit, or character.[1]

Before we can deal with how you are aging, before we can look to the future, yours and ours, we must first go back in time . . . way back. Because, as much as we like to think that we're all unique individuals (and we are), we have much—enormous amounts in fact—in common. This can be both alarming and comforting, but it's nonetheless true. We must understand the source of that commonality and, understanding it, use that understanding to make our journey to better health and aging a more valuable and productive experience.

As we look to our ancestors to explain our commonality, please note that I am not advocating in any way a return to a pre-Industrial Revolution society. What I am advocating is an awareness of what we need to be healthy and age well, and that we begin to creatively reintroduce these authentically human elements into our individual lives and into our society.

CHAPTER 1

WHERE ARE WE NOW?
HOW DID WE GET HERE?

Every man is a quotation from all his ancestors.
—RALPH WALDO EMERSON

We are a marvel. Many trillions of cells all functioning as one magnificent being. Short, tall, male, female, dark, light, blue eyes, brown eyes, happy, morose, athletic, intellectual, quick, or slow—we are human, *Homo sapiens*, "knowing man," the only living species in the *Homo* genus. Our ancestors who most looked like us originated in Africa about 200,000 years ago. If we go back further, to ancestors who looked more like our primate cousins (the DNA of these current cousins is 98 percent identical to ours), it's four to eight million years ago. And if we consider other mammals that may not look like us but with whom we share much—from how we procreate and nurture offspring to how we respond to threats—well, now we're talking several hundred million years.

Max Delbrück, the Nobel Prize–winning biophysicist, tells us that any living cell carries with it the experience of a billion years of experimentation by its ancestors. These ancestors gave us much more than a family tree. The very things that make us distinctly human were unknowingly tested and perfected by them. The successful ones passed down that success to us. How our hearts and brains and lungs and kidneys and guts work, how our bodies respond to certain foods, how we learn, what we need to feel secure and thrive—all these things were refined by our ancestors and passed down to us. These are our *authentic* traits, in other words, the ones that are truly human, forged by eons of our species' history, shared by all of us, and durable over time despite marked changes in how we live today. You might say our ancestors worked out the bugs and that we are the prize of all those millions of years of trials: a complex, thinking, adaptable and rational being who dominates the world.

And we do dominate the world, right? Sure, our brains and our ability to manipulate our environment allow us to push our weight around and walk with a swagger amongst our fellow creatures. However, we humans can get a bit carried away with ourselves. Jonas Salk saw our existence in perspective. "If all the insects were to disappear from the earth," he said, "within fifty years all other forms of life would end. But if all human beings were to disappear from the earth, within fifty years all other forms of life would flourish." As we have developed the tools to better evaluate the cognitive and emotional capabilities of our fellow mammals, especially primates, we are finding that many higher-level skills and social interactions are not unique to us humans.

Still, consumed with ourselves or not, we are indeed a masterpiece. A being able to communicate complex ideas, to build cities and washing machines and airplanes and space stations and iPads, to write books, to discover the human genome, to invent bubble gum; the tip of the earth's pyramid of living things; the final product of a very long assembly line of trial and error, success and failure, and system refinement. But there's a catch.

With these superpowers we have transformed the earth. In just the blink of a geologic eye, we have moved from caves to skyscrapers, from walking to Segways, from combing the earth for roots and berries and nuts to McDonald's, from spears to nukes, from conversation to texting, from gazing into a fire to multitasking. The speed of that change has been something the earth has never seen before and it is ever accelerating.

Yet our bodies are slackers when it comes to this rate of change. Our physiologic systems do not change that quickly. What we require to be healthy and flourish is not very different from what our ancestors required. We are essentially a 2.0-version human in the 10.0 world we have created. This is readily apparent when we attempt to explain why we are captivated by campfires, storytelling, and even drum circles; why green is a color that soothes us; why we crave to be part of a group and yet are suspicious of strangers; why we are fascinated by animals; why loud noises still startle us and a walk in the woods relaxes most of us. In 1979, René Dubois, in the introduction to Norman Cousins's *Anatomy of an Illness*, wrote, "Even under the most urbanized conditions, we retain the genetic constitution of our Stone Age ancestors and therefore can never be completely adapted."[1] Jon Kabat-Zinn, who developed the Mindfulness-Based Stress Reduction program, calls us "analog creatures in a digital world."[2]

This failure of our bodies to adapt at the same rate as we have developed our civilization has resulted in a maladaptation, particularly in areas of health and behavior. This maladaptation has our bodies functioning in a "foreign" world, has our bodies and minds desperately seeking what they need to be healthy and functioning at their best but finding it more and more difficult in a world rapidly moving away from the one our ancestors adapted to eons ago. Joan Vinge, author of the award-winning *The Snow Queen*, tells us that "humans are upsetting a fragile balance that their own human ancestors established."[3] Jared Diamond, UCLA professor and renowned author of *Collapse* and *Guns, Germs and Steel*, writes in his latest book, *The World Until Yesterday*, "In some respects we moderns are misfits: our bodies and our practices now face conditions different from those under which they evolved, and to which they became adapted." [4] And Robert Wright, an evolutionary psychologist, states in his compelling book *The Moral Animal*, "We are not designed to stand on crowded subway platforms, or to live in suburbs next door to people we never talk to, or to get hired or fired, or to watch the evening news. This disjunction between the contexts of our design (our ancestral environment) and of our lives is probably responsible for much psychopathology, as well as much suffering."[5]

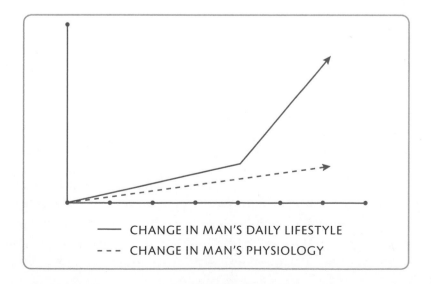

— CHANGE IN MAN'S DAILY LIFESTYLE

- - - CHANGE IN MAN'S PHYSIOLOGY

The way we were

We've all heard it, from our grandparents, or parents, or two old gentlemen talking on a bench. It usually starts out with "In my day, we . . ." and you can fill in the rest.

"In my day, we walked to school in snow up to our waist," one says.

The other responds, "We didn't even have boots for our feet."

And the final word: "Feet? You had feet?"

It's a caricature, yes, but tales of tougher times are not far-fetched when it comes to our ancestors who lived millennia before us. Remember, these are the ancestors from whom we've inherited most of the physiology, instincts, needs, likes, and dislikes that we think are our own preferences but that are in fact the result of a long history of survival and necessity. So we wonder. How was the life of our ancestors different from ours? Does it matter?

It has only been about ten generations, 250 years, since the Industrial Revolution began to change our world drastically. For four hundred generations before that, approximately ten thousand years, we lived primarily in agricultural societies where we pretty much stayed put, raised crops, domesticated animals, and reaped a dividend of a higher survival and overall quality of life. But for perhaps as much as *72,000 generations or more* before that, we were hunter-gatherers. When our distinctly human characteristics were developing, we were essentially nomadic and tightly bound in small groups and villages. Put another way, if all of the time humans have been on earth was one year, then the Industrial Revolution would have occurred in the last hour of the year, our agrarian period would be less than *two days*, and the hunter-gatherer period would be 363 days! Can we be so arrogant as to think that what we are today, psychologically, physically, instinctually—and what we need to be healthy, happy; what we need to age well—was determined in the last few centuries? In the last few decades? In the last few years? Or weeks? Clearly the environment in which our ancestors lived had a huge impact not only on them but also on modern-day humans, their relatively recent offspring.

So it becomes crucial to our own understanding of who we are and what we need to be healthy and age well that we break out the human family photo album and carefully look at the environment of our esteemed ancestors. What was life like for these hunter-gatherers? What food did they eat? How did they spend their days? What behaviors allowed them to survive and eventually bring us into existence? What were the conditions under which we humans became who we are?

A Day in the Life of Your Great (Times Many Thousands) Grandfather

He rose with the sun that brought light and heat to the day. There was no time, only the passing of the light, full moons, the repetition of seasons, and the birth and death of living things around him. This was the nature of things, and he was at peace with it. He stoked the embers from last night's fire, added wood from the pile the children had gathered, and brought flames to life. The tribe was all rising with him. There was work to do. If they had been successful finding food in yesterday's light, they all gathered and ate the rewards: the nuts, berries, fruits, and wild vegetables. One of the children had found the carcass of a dead deer, and a group of other children had collected what the predator and birds had left. That was a treat they had all enjoyed by last night's fire while the child proudly told the story of finding it.

As the sun arced over the sky, your ancestor and most of the others walked, looking for food. Since they were traveling farther and farther for food, they would soon move the shelters again. The light was getting short, it was getting colder, and they would move to the place where there were small animals and more roots, and shelter from the winds.

Most of his children had lived and he liked watching them contribute more to the tribe. They were raised by the entire tribe and responded to all who guided them, particularly the older women. Their mothers had all lived through childbirth also and were some of the strongest walkers and most successful food finders and gatherers in the tribe.

When an event happened to one of them, it was recognized by all: a birth, a death, a rite of passage, the discovery of a better food area, good weather. They came together and would often sing and dance as a group. The group was the most important thing. Whatever your ancestor could do that would help the tribe, the whole group, that was what he must do. He remembered from his childhood a man who'd been exiled for hoarding food during a meager time. He would never do such a thing.

After spending all the light time walking and gathering food, he looked forward to being with everyone else around the fire, hearing stories of the old and young, but particularly the stories of the elders. He was close to being an elder himself, and tried to learn as much as possible from the current elders so that he could tell the stories of their history and keep the tribe safe and thriving when they depended on him for guidance. He had learned to observe: to notice any changes in the behavior of their brother and sister animals, fish, and birds that might indicate a threat or availability of food; to watch the clouds, winds, and temperatures to predict storms. He was one of the most successful in the tribe at finding food. He could build or find shelter whenever the tribe needed it. These were the skills that were most important for the survival of all, and he was respected by all and would never let the tribe down.

A Peek into Our Past

We can get more than a speculative view of the hunter-gatherer environment through the observations of anthropologists like Hugh Brody and Marjorie Shostak, both of whom lived in current-day hunter-gatherer societies. Brody, a writer, anthropologist, and filmmaker, lived with the Inuit in the Arctic and with the salmon-fishing tribes of the Canadian Northwest. In his book *The Other Side of Eden*, Brody dispels myths of hunter-gatherer societies as primitive and brutish, nomadic in the sense that they were never connected to place: "The thing about being with the Inuit is that you have a sense of being with the most gracious, most generous, most sophisticated of human beings. So far from being simple, they are very, very rich and complex." Likewise, he describes their culture as respectful to both the planet and its people. Rather than having a drifter mentality, "hunter-gatherers are completely committed to one place because their success depends on their knowledge of the one place and their knowledge is not transferable."[6]

Marjorie Shostak lived with the !Kung San people of the Kalahari Desert in southwestern Africa and focused on the status of women in this hunter-gatherer society, concluding that !Kung San women had higher status and autonomy than women in Western cultures because of their food contributions.[7] Rather than describing primitive people, the observations of these authors give us a rich look into our human mirror and help us understand why we are the way we are. What it is, in fact, that makes us human. Whether we can attribute the characteristics of modern-day hunter-gather populations to our distant ancestors might be debatable, but I believe most would concede that they are culturally as closely connected to our ancestral past as any other group of humans currently living.

Even a cursory review of the literature about current hunter-gatherer cultures leads one to make some general conclusions that are both surprising and revealing.

Hunter-gatherer cultures . . .

- are egalitarian, with women having social equality with men
- are happy, with people laughing freely
- are nonviolent
- have strong safety nets that support the old, the disabled, the young, the unfortunate
- are inclusive, with no one marginalized except as punishment for an offense
- have sharing as a core characteristic
- are in harmony with the earth, relying on renewable resources

Although today's hunter-gatherer cultures are doubtless affected in some ways by modern-day civilization, it seems rational to assume that these cultures reflect, at least to some degree, and to a degree much more than our current society, the culture of our distant ancestors and—because of the sheer predominance of this culture in our overall history—the environment to which we as humans are most adapted.

Our Distant Roots, in Summary

So, what generalizations can we make about our ancestors? First, most of their activities were geared toward survival: their own, that of their tribe, and without their being aware of it, that of our very species. They worked hard for food. In most environments, even when food was plentiful, it took much work to gather and transport it back to the rest of the tribe or village. Whether gathering or hunting, obtaining food required much greater expenditure of energy than it does today. *Our ancestors moved*—a lot—in search of food and shelter. Because food could not be preserved, there was a tendency to eat heavily when it was available. Even though it was very rare, our ancestors preferred high-fat food, because it was calorie rich and able to sustain them for when food was not available—a trait that causes difficulty today. Their diets consisted of mainly fruits, wild vegetables and grains, nuts, fish, and the occasional meat from a small animal or the leftovers from a predator's kill. Remembering locations for food and water was a critical skill (which explains why our memory for images and locations is much better than for numbers and names). They ate often, foraging for whatever food was available. Sugar, other than that found naturally in foods, was foreign to their physiology.

Exposure to the elements was a major concern, especially in northern latitudes. Infant deaths were very common, and conception and nurturing of the young were a major focus of the entire group, yet they could not preclude the mother's role in gathering and preparing food. Basically, it took a village to survive and thrive and it was primarily the older adults who cared for children (accounting, I believe, for the near mystical relationship between grandparents and children). Everyone had a role in this survival scenario. Everyone had a place, a status, and a familiarity with all others in the band. There was a social compact: I help you and you help me. Sharing was core to how our ancestors interacted with each other. Helping others in the group was not viewed as a service but was expected. (My friend Alison McReynolds spent time in Mauritania and was surprised to learn there was no word for *volunteering* in the language of the village people she worked with.) There was great respect for others in the tribe or village but a suspicion of others not in their tribe, a xenophobia that made sense given that each tribe was competing for the limited resources they needed to survive.

Actions that benefited the individual over the greater good of the tribe were considered heinous and could result in banishment, the ultimate punishment and an almost guaranteed death sentence. Members of the group, tribe, and even village had little concept of themselves as single entities in the world, but only as part of group. That group, in fact, gave them their only chance for survival.

Time had little meaning beyond the seasons, the cycle of the moon, and availability of food. Our ancestors were intimately tied to the rhythms of nature. They woke not to alarm clocks but to the light. They spent dark hours, when work was not possible, telling stories, propagating their own history, usually around a fire. Communication was oral and face-to-face, even before language was known and certainly after. Stress was similar to that experienced by their mammal cousins: It came from the hunt or being hunted, the potential threat from strangers, storms, famine. When these threats weren't present, their lives were peaceful and in harmony with nature.

Infections and accidents were the primary killers. Average life expectancy then, and for most of time man has been on earth up until recent millennia, was two, perhaps three decades. Infections and accidents or childhood diseases killed most—and usually fairly quickly.

In today's hunter-gatherer cultures, the older in the tribe are not marginalized but rather celebrated, and it would make sense that it would be similar with our ancestors. Old age was rare and therefore revered, respected, and associated with high stature. Life on the move was harsh, however, and any reverence for the older was tempered by the reality of this life. Simone de Beauvoir, in her 1970 book *The Coming of Age*,[8] bore witness to this harshness toward elders when they could no longer move with the group and therefore threatened the survival of all. Despite these rare instances of elder pruning, living long was a great accomplishment and lucky indeed was a tribe that had an elder to advise them on the best course of action when the tribe was challenged. In fact, older adults had a key role in the overall functioning of the tribe. This role was viewed as a responsibility, neither optional nor insignificant. It would essentially remain this way in subsequent societies, until the mid-eighteenth century.

So, we have these early humans, who looked a lot like us—our family tree. We are happy indeed that they survived in a very difficult environment. Had they not, of course, I wouldn't be writing this and you wouldn't be reading. We would not exist. In fact, everything they did had a survival purpose: having *connections with others* helped each survive; constantly *moving* and searching for food kept them from starving; having a *purpose* that involved the greater good of the tribe helped the group survive; behavior that fostered the *conception and nurturing of children* helped them survive as a tribe and as a race. And so these traits were deeply embedded in our human brains as instinctual preferences. And although our world today is radically different, we maintain the basic makeup that helped them adapt to and survive in their world.

We Settle Down

And then, approximately ten thousand years ago, we began to gather in villages as we started to grow crops and domesticate animals. We became agrarian societies and were now able to stay in place. We exchanged the nomadic *lifestyle* for more permanent and effective shelters, the increased availability of food, and more types of food, with more meat and cultivated crops. What did not change appreciably was the tight social fabric of the group, the social compact, the high level of physical movement, and the necessity to work together for the common good— i.e., a harvest that would sustain the village. Your great (times four hundred) grandmother worked in the fields or tended animals most of the day until she was older and then was in charge of the youngest children, who could not yet work in the fields. The harvest was the most important concern of the entire village, and she had an important role to play. To not do her part was unthinkable.

Hunter-gatherer
- Small groups/tribes
- Frequent moving/nomadic
- Skillful/nimble/efficient/adaptable
- Food sources wild/scarce
- Diet of fruits/wild vegetables/nuts/wild grains/fish/some small game
- Less prone to disease

Agrarian
- Larger groups/towns
- Stable/permanent shelters
- More rooted in place
- Food more plentiful
- Diet of more meat/grains
- More susceptible to infectious disease

And then, after approximately four hundred generations of this agrarian culture, and only ten generations ago, the Industrial Revolution arrived and everything changed—truly everything. Virtually every aspect of the daily life of most humans was altered by this massive shift in how we humans lived. Humans found themselves in environments very foreign to what they, their parents, and their earlier ancestors had experienced—not only fish out of water, but fish thrown into a cesspool.

A Day in the Life of Your Great-(Times Ten) Grandfather

He rose before dawn, as did the whole family. The sounds of his neighbors also rising early was insurance against sleeping too long. To be late was to be jobless; to be jobless was to be destitute. Breakfast was meager but filling. He left the apartment with his two sons, twelve and ten, who had been able to get jobs picking up scraps of material. His wife would be sewing all day, repairing the clothing of their neighbors for money or food. He and his sons walked in the dark, alongside other men and sons who lived nearby but whom he didn't know very well. They punched in at the tin factory and began their twelve-hour shift. If he was lucky he could get a sixteen-hour shift occasionally. They had it better than other workers. They had three breaks, two for the bathroom and another fifteen minutes to eat the lunch his wife had packed. He wouldn't see his boys until the shift was over.

This ancestor was a very good worker, turning out higher numbers than others and therefore never getting close to being fired for low output. He stood in one place all day punching holes in pieces of metal. He had come close to missing his quota when he had influenza last year. Many of the workers in his area had been fired. Many had died of influenza. In fact, they had lost many of their friends—fathers, mothers, children—as the disease spread rapidly through the neighborhood. He was terrified when his three-year-old daughter began coughing. He had her seen by a midwife, who had told them to boil water to make steam for her to breath. She had lost weight but survived.

They were saving the money from his wife's sewing and hoped someday to join his brother in Toledo, who said wages were higher and shifts shorter. Maybe they could rent a larger house with a yard. He was convinced they could do this if he could stay healthy.

At the end of the shift a whistle blew and he met his sons at the gate and they walked home quietly with the same group from the morning. Dinner would be ready. They would sit at the table talking. His wife would do some lessons with the boys, hoping they would become good enough readers to get steady jobs when they were older. Sleep came early and easy after a long day of monotonous work.

A PBS special on Andrew Carnegie described the even more challenging life of steel workers, who labored every day of the week in twelve-hour shifts. They got one holiday a year: the Fourth of July. The TV program highlighted the workers' perspectives on their jobs in the steel mills: "Hard! I guess it's hard," said a laborer at the Homestead mill. "I lost forty pounds the first three months I came into this business. It sweats the life out of a man." . . . "You don't notice any old men here," said a Homestead laborer in 1894. "The long hours, the strain, and the sudden changes of temperature use a man up." Sociologist John A. Fitch called it "old age at forty."[9]

A Peek Into Our More Recent Past

Postindustrial life, then, represented a dramatic shift from the hunter-gatherer lifestyle and even from the more recent agrarian lifestyle that preceded industrialization.

Postindustrial urban cultures . . .

- were highly stratified, with few haves and many have-nots
- were grueling, with little time for recreation
- were marked by class violence and competition for resources
- were isolating and marked by poverty, with essentially no safety nets
- considered the old and disabled useless and a burden
- were removed from nature and associated with environmental pollution

Our More Recent Roots, Summing Up

With the industrialization of Europe and America, we moved from our rural homes to cities. Work now was tedious, done under noisy and dirty conditions, and determined by the clock. And not only work was affected: Meals, school, sleep, recreation were all tied to the work clock. Shifts were ten to twelve—even sixteen—hours with few breaks. Factory smoke frequently blocked the sun, and cities were gloomy and dark. Stress rose as the demand for production drove employers to demand more and more from workers. Although there was some banding together of ethnic groups or former village members, for the most part families found themselves on their own, with no village to rely on if health or finances took a bad turn. Individuals had to provide for themselves and their families. Women whose husbands died found themselves destitute and out of options. Income rose, but so did the cost of food, shelter, and basic necessities. Illness or injury could result in loss of work, with devastating consequences. Children were exploited as a cheap labor source.

Diseases of urbanization, such as cholera, influenza, and tuberculosis, killed or incapacitated huge segments of the population. The early Industrial Revolution saw a dip in life expectancy, most prominently among children and factory workers. By the mid-nineteenth century, however, populations were growing, and average life expectancy increased due to better access to regular food. When Louis Pasteur and Robert Koch formulated the germ theory of disease and Pasteur developed the first vaccines in the second half of the nineteenth century, lifespan increased significantly. In 1855, Dr. John Snow was able to pinpoint a particular water supply, the Broad Street pump in London, as the source of the cholera epidemic that was sweeping through the city and killing tens of thousands.[10] By removing the handle to that pump, he was able to stop the epidemic. In 1867, English surgeon Joseph Lister championed the use of carbolic acid as an antiseptic, significantly reducing the likelihood of infection and death associated with surgery, and in 1908, the first city-wide treatment of water with chlorine began in Jersey City, New Jersey.

Life expectancy at the end of the nineteenth century in the United States was still approximately age forty-nine, but these discoveries, which provided safe water, infection-reduced surgery and childbirth, vaccines, and, eventually, in 1928, penicillin, began to increase longevity dramatically. In fact, in the twentieth century alone, lifespan increased more than it had since the Bronze Age. We were bright. We were beautiful. We were the rulers of the earth. Maybe we would live forever.

The way we are

Today, we live longer than our ancestors of any era. We're able to travel anywhere on the globe and even into space. We produce and transport any commodity needed: food, cars, electronics, and clothing. We rarely die of infectious disease, and can replace hearts, kidneys, shoulders, knees, and hips. Yes, we have come a long way from our humble roots as a species.

We awake in temperature-controlled houses, have ready access to showers and baths. Our breakfast is in the refrigerator or cupboard, or at the nearest restaurant. It's whatever we want and as much as we want. We sit and eat. We sit in our cars and drive to work. Many of us sit at work, peering into computer screens or talking on telephones. We spend long hours looking at screens: computers, iPhones, televisions, GPS devices, games. We have tens, even hundreds, of friends, but rarely touch their hands, or look into their eyes, or sit peacefully hearing their stories. We use our cars as transporters, offices, and image enhancers. Fast, calorie-rich food is everywhere and affordable, ready to pick up at the end of a drive-through line.

Our time-saving devices allow us to rush about and accomplish so much more. We move fast on freeways while we order a pizza. We text a friend while talking to another. We attend meetings and read texts and emails while the speaker is telling us how to be more efficient. We have devices that do our math, look up any known fact, correct our spelling, and type what we say. Our children are musicians, and athletes, and dancers, and busy. Many of us have nannies, and landscapers, and painters, and personal assistants, and life coaches. We can drive through restaurants, car washes, banks, coffee houses, and pharmacies. And yes, we have pills to make us feel better, or get thinner, or sleep better, or to prevent allergies or colds. If we're feeling sluggish, we can get more energy from the contents of a can or bottle.

We are efficient machines, able to accomplish more and more if we get the right tools, and if we just go a little faster, or sleep less, or just try harder.

Mulch, Steve, and the Gym

We have lived in this evolved society our whole lives, and as a result, we are less than objective, even blind, when it comes to the way we now live. So, let me tell you about my last twenty-four hours. Yesterday I spent many hours preparing my flower and ornamental grass beds and then spreading mulch. It was work I wasn't used to. But I resolved to be mindful about this work rather than complain or think about what I would do when I was done. Along the way of spreading this mulch, something happened. A switch flipped and I became very aware of the sweet smell of the mulch, of its warmth. And I was pleased with these feelings. This was not tedious work. In fact, being able to see the fruits of my work, something immediate, concrete, and visual, gave me surprising, pleasant sensations. My work, preventing disease, is rewarding work, but you rarely get a glimpse of the result, and almost never immediately.

And as I spread the mulch I could feel my leg, arm, back, and abdominal muscles moving, contracting, relaxing. I was aware of a feeling of optimism, of overall physical well-being, much like the endorphin rush we get when we exert ourselves physically. And I thought, why should this happen?

Our ancestors had to work hard, and if there were no reward other than survival, why would mankind persist? There had to be more immediate gratification, hence the myriad of neurotransmitters that flood us after running a race, or building a fence, or mulching a flower bed. And my response was more than physical. Mentally there was a relief from my normal mind chatter about what I had to do that week, or problems at work, or what Jack meant by that remark, or how long I could hold off on buying a new car. This relief provided me a feeling of peace and mental well-being. I became more attentive to the smell and feel of the mulch. I was a happy camper.

My neighbor Steve drove by as I was working. He laughed and said, "You know, there are people who do that. Why are you doing it? I had someone come and it was done in no time." As he drove away, I thought about his remark. I would miss the near spiritual experience (it hadn't started that way, but as I grew more mindful, it became so much more). I would miss the pleasing sensation of my body in motion. I would miss the sense of accomplishment. I would miss the feeling I would have over the next year as I looked out on my lawn. I'm sure it makes financial sense for Steve to not spread his own mulch, but what he's missing—a connection with those who came before us, and to what makes us human—is priceless.

Today, although a little sore, I went to the fitness center. As I pedaled away on a recumbent bicycle, the woman next to me was also pedaling—and texting, and reading, and listening to music.

Now, the attitudes and actions of people like Steve and this woman at the gym aren't uncommon. They are, however, at least for me, on this day, a litmus test of our society's separation from its roots. Considering the lives of our ancestors (the word *lifestyle* doesn't seem to fit), our current lifestyle represents an ever-growing gap between their world and our own. It's progress, yes, but a kind of progress our bodies cannot adapt to, and we are suffering because of it.

Modern Man's Dilemma

Yes, it is true that average life expectancy increased more in the twentieth century alone than it had since the Bronze Age, but this is more a matter of knowledge and technology breakthroughs than any change in how our bodies function. In fact, living longer has presented us with health, quality-of-life, and societal challenges we are totally unprepared to manage.

When we look at our lives today, we see that they are radically different from those of our ancestors. Time is king. Time is money. Idleness is the evil empire. We multitask—no, we are *obsessed* with multitasking. Technology and societal values allow us to believe we are indeed effective because we're driving, drinking our coffee, talking on the phone, thinking of the upcoming meeting, and railing against the jerk who just cut in front of us. We spend a large proportion of our daily lives sitting. We are texting and emailing in prodigious numbers and "friending" or "connecting" with people we've never meet or never will. All this results in us being everywhere but where we are. Our area of focus is expanded at the expense of our sense of ourselves in *this moment*, the only place where we truly experience our existence. Our sense of accomplishment is enhanced at the expense of our sense of well-being.

We are left with a feeling of being alone in a hostile world, and consequently we tenaciously fight for our piece of the pie, for our personal rights, for what is good for us and our immediate family. Our purpose, for a good part of our lives, revolves around our personal advancement: wealth, prestige, and comfort. We vote for those who promise to give us what we consider important, even at the expense of what is good for a greater number. The end result of this survivalist and self-absorbed approach to life is a chronic, continuous, consuming, and killing stress. When we fail to perceive ourselves as part of all life, or a member of our human race, or part of a country, or part of a village, we become isolated in a way our ancestors never knew, and we are the worse for it. Many of our illnesses are those of maladaptation: exposure to a world of food, to chemicals, and to a time-obsessed, noisy, high-tech culture our body systems are not yet equipped to deal with. We suffer from chronic disease, spending large portions of our now longer lives impaired in some way. We are so much better off than our ancestors . . . and yet we are not.

Robin Wright sums up our modern plight in *The Moral Animal*: "We live in cities and suburbs and watch TV and drink beer, all the while being pushed and pulled by feelings designed to propagate our genes in a small hunter-gatherer population. It's no wonder that people often seem not to be pursuing any particular goal—happiness, inclusive fitness, whatever—very successfully."[11]

And what about being old?

As for what it is like to be old today versus when your great, great, great (times a few thousand) grandparents walked the earth, the disparity is stark. First of all, older people aren't rare. With average life expectancy nearly doubling in the last century, and with eight to ten thousand boomers turning sixty-five every day in the United States, elderhood is more common today. That said, elders have no established role in society. No necessary, established expectation or responsibility. They are programmed into a marginal position of leisure and entitlement, essentially invisible in the media unless the object of ageist humor or described as part of an overall societal financial liability. The time-honored advice to "respect your elders" is rarely heard and less often practiced. This all sounds grim, markedly unlike the experience of our hunter-gatherer or agrarian ancestors, but is entirely consistent with a postindustrial, production-oriented society.

Let's now outline some of the biggest differences between humanity's past and present.

Ancestral/Preindustrial

Society
- egalitarian
- mostly content
- basically nonviolent
- strong social safety nets
- inclusive/high sense of belonging
- sharing as a core characteristic
- harmony with the earth

Lifestyle
- highly physical
- strong social connection
- strong sense of place/purpose
- diet based on plants, fruits, nuts, fish, occasional meat/limited overall calories/obesity rare
- little chronic stress

Status of older adults

- essential role as advisors
- valued
- non-sedentary
- supported by society
- critical role in social fabric
- viewed as uncommon and cultural treasures

Postindustrial/Modern

Society

- stratified economically
- high stress
- regimented work/recreation
- violence common
- time dominant
- limited social/financial safety nets
- high alienation and isolation
- more removed from nature/pollution more common

Lifestyle

- more commonly sedentary
- traditional social connection less common
- roles based on occupation or parental status
- mobile
- diet of calorie-rich food/less plant-based/additives common
- high chronic stress

Status of older adults

- no established role
- viewed as societal liability
- more sedentary/chronic disease common
- marginalized/isolated with growing age
- size of population growing rapidly

In short, we are living under conditions radically different from the ones our species has lived under for 99 percent of the time we've walked the earth, and from our basic, authentic-needs point of view, much of this change doesn't represent progress.

We are what we are

We are an aging nation. There's nothing we can do about it. The huge birth rate after World War II and through the Korean War and the rocking fifties—from 1946 to 1964—produced 76 million children, who are now turning sixty-five at a rate of nearly ten thousand every day. These and other trends are changing us as a people and as a nation. The Population Reference Bureau summed up these trends back in 2004: "The US is getting bigger, older, and more diverse."[12] (By "bigger," the report means "more populated," although obesity is certainly another trend.) More diversity will indeed present challenges to us as a nation, particularly when some persist in thinking we are a static mix of people, mostly of European background.

Ken Dychtwald, a psychologist, gerontologist, and prolific author, began speaking of this dramatic bigger-older-and-more-diverse transformation of our society in the 1970s, calling it the "Age Wave," a term that serves as both the title of his company and the title of his 1990 book.[13] The Age Wave Dr. Dychtwald speaks of is not only the result of the post–World War II birth increase but also of the increasing life expectancy and declining birth rates of the last few decades. He foresaw that the aging of our society would have profound effects on nearly every aspect of our lives, with "no business, family or home [working] tomorrow as it does today."[14]

Dr. Dychtwald's predictions were spot on. Not only are we proportionally and numerically older than any society in human history, but we have, in the last hundred years or so, made a radical shift from one thing we as humans have believed and valued for centuries, even eons. Namely, we have marginalized our older population, placing them on the fringes of what we now consider important.

Basically, we act like, and therefore believe, that older adults are a societal responsibility; productive years are behind them; they are in a recreation or entitlement mode; they are cranky and demanding. Nowhere is our low value of older adults more evident than in the media. At a minimum, television and movies portray older adults in a manner that does not evoke respect. At its worst, older adults are the object of mocking humor and condescending pity. Perhaps this attitude stems from a utilitarian view of people as workers that began with the Industrial Revolution and has carried over into the digital age, or from the related phenomenon of older adults turning their back on salaried employment as soon as possible and adopting a recreational "fully retired" lifestyle. Or perhaps it's just an accurate depiction of the result of our marginalizing public policies. In any case, it will come as a surprise to many that this less-than-flattering view of older adults is a new phenomenon.

Dychtwald reminds us in his book *Age Power*: "For most of history, in fact, it was maturity that was prized. Until relatively recently, the old, more than any other group, controlled power, assumed leadership, and set the example for others. In the early centuries of American history, in nearly every aspect of community, family, and work life, old people reigned. Only during the twentieth century have they temporarily been knocked to the mat, viewed largely as a social burden.[15] Dr. Dychtwald also believes that this situation will shift, and that belief is the basis for his prediction of "profound changes" made in *Age Wave*.

We will return to predictions later, but first, let's discuss the basis for these predictions.

CHAPTER 2

WHAT WE KNOW NOW

*Death is not the greatest loss in life. The greatest loss
is what dies inside us while we live.*
—NORMAN COUSINS

The cat's out of the bag and there's no going back. Your grandmother's belief that how she aged was primarily determined by genes and a little bit of luck, well, that belief has gone the way of the eight-track player. The fact is, we can no longer blame our parents for our aging experience. In 1984, the MacArthur Foundation assembled the Research Network on Successful Aging and began what was to be a seminal study on aging. Jonas Salk, the foundation's most famous board member, had challenged them to study the successes and not the negative aspects of aging. Their findings changed our understanding of aging forever, jolting us from our Dark Age attitude into a revolutionary new perspective of this common human experience.

This historic study clearly proved that *how we age is mostly up to us,* and it rocked our stereotypes of aging to the core, challenging us as a society to rethink long-standing assumptions; forcing us to reevaluate approaches to healthcare, senior living, retirement, education, and even recreation. It also threw down a gauntlet, a moral imperative, to rid ourselves of what Dr. Robert Butler labeled "ageism" in his 1975 book, *Why Survive?: Being Old in America.*[1] Ageism is age discrimination, which commonly fosters a stereotype or notion of aging as mostly about decline. With the MacArthur Study findings, such a notion was now no longer tenable.

It's all about compression

The MacArthur Study findings were clear: 70 percent of the physical difference and 50 percent of the intellectual difference between those who age in the usual way and those who age more successfully were due to lifestyle, the choices we make every day.

So, we ask, what does all this mean? If I age successfully, just what does that look like? What happens if I don't live this lifestyle the MacArthur Study described? Do I age unsuccessfully? Drs. Rowe and Kahn are very clear about this, and our aging curve helps us to understand their guidance. Aging in the "usual" way is pictured in figure 2 as the solid line: an aging experience in which we are born, grow to maturity, and then at some point, because most diseases that kill us now are chronic diseases (rather than the acute diseases that ended the lives of our ancestors), begin a period of decline. This decline can now dominate a larger and larger portion of our lifespan because we've learned how to manage—yet not cure—chronic diseases such as heart disease, lung disease, arthritis, diabetes, and even cancer. Successful aging, on the other hand, depicted as the dotted line, is associated with maintaining abilities for a longer time, declining more slowly, and remaining minimally impaired despite advancing age.

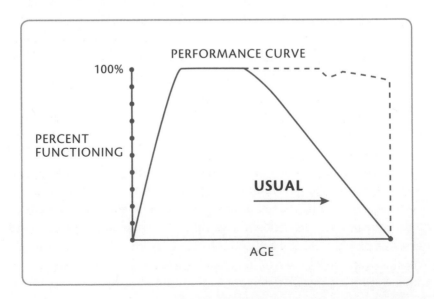

It is clear from this curve that since lifestyle choices are associated with a more successful aging experience, such choices influence not only the quality of our life but also the quality of our death. Since life expectancy has upper limits, the longer we can stay at high levels of function, the more likely that the "terminal event," as we say in medicine, will be short. This is called *compression of morbidity*, and it is the key to dealing with the dramatic demographic shift we are experiencing worldwide. Dr. James Fries introduced this concept in a keynote address to the National Academy of Science's Institute of Medicine in 1982.[2] Compression of morbidity essentially means that the time we are sick at the end of our life is short: Rather than living the later phase of our life according to the predictions of those who associate aging with decline (my friend and colleague Dr. Bill Thomas calls these people "declinists"), we can indeed choose another route, a higher road more under our control even at the road's end. According to the MacArthur research, my autumn leaf analogy—in other words, dying short—is possible!

Consider the final chapter in two men's lives. Andrew is eighty-five years old and on his deathbed. For the last year, he has been bedridden in a nursing home, too weak to sit up. Three years ago, he fell and broke his hip. After nearly six months in bed he was able to walk minimally with a walker. Ten years ago he had a stroke that paralyzed his right side and left him unable to speak. After a year of rehabilitation, he was able to walk and speak, but with difficulty. Fifteen years ago, he had a mild heart attack, caused, his doctors said, by his long-standing adult-onset diabetes, which had in turn been brought on by his obesity.

Harold, eighty-six years old, is tragically killed by a drunk driver while bicycling in Spain. The week before, he watched the running of the bulls in Pamplona, something he had wanted to see most of his life. He had been on a month-long trip with his wife and granddaughter through France, Portugal, and Morocco. He'd taken the vacation after finishing his third book on American history, a topic he had pursued avidly after his retirement from his accounting business.

Two stories. One of "usual" aging, in that it is a story of decline not unexpected in our society. The other of vitality and purpose right up to the last moments. One with almost two decades of impairment, dependence, and lower quality of life. The other with a very brief end. Both gone, but with a dramatic difference in the last phase of life. If you could pick between the two, it's obvious which you would choose. And now we know we can. But do we?

Live long, die short: Why not?

OK. So, in a nutshell: We can live a longer, higher-quality life that ends in a short time (like fall foliage dropping off the tree) without the pain, expense, anxiety, and burden to our families. Do I have any takers?

Of course I do. Who wouldn't want this? And luckily, *we* are the biggest factor in making this happen. Yet you wouldn't think so when you look at the numbers. Despite the fact that we're pretty much in the driver's seat as to how we age, when you look at the major causes of death, they are chronic, slow-decline, "I've lost control of my life"–type conditions. There's no dropping off the tree with most of them.

Here are, according to the Centers for Disease Control, the major causes of death in the United States in 2010:

- Heart disease: 597,689
- Cancer: 574,743
- Chronic lower respiratory diseases: 138,080
- Stroke (cerebrovascular diseases): 129,476
- Accidents (unintentional injuries): 120,859
- Alzheimer's disease: 83,494
- Diabetes: 69,071
- Nephritis, nephrotic syndrome, and nephrosis: 50,476
- Influenza and pneumonia: 50,097
- Intentional self-harm (suicide): 38,364[3]

At least six, and some may argue all, of these causes of death are modifiable by lifestyle and life choices. We can avoid them, have them for a shorter period of our lives, or have them with less impairment. The MacArthur Study removed the veil of fatalism and impotency from these conditions. And here's more good news from the MacArthur research: *It is never too late to make a difference*, to change the slope of our own aging curve. Even when life throws you one of its inevitable curveballs and you find yourself having lost some of your abilities, it is absolutely possible, and in fact necessary, that you respond in a deliberate way, with the knowledge of what it takes to prove the declinists wrong, and halt your slide by stabilizing what you do have, or regaining some, or all, of what you've lost. Lamenting your loss, beating your breast over it, or accepting it as part of your inevitable decline is inviting a trip further down the slide.

In fact, the whole new area of study of Epigenetics tells us that our lifestyle may very well be able to switch genes on and off, making it quite possible that disease-causing genes may never be expressed. This could very well be the cellular explanation for why lifestyle is indeed the major determinant in how we age rather than our genes.

We now have a picture of aging that is empowering, in that each of us has a major input in what kind of older adult we will be, how independent or dependent, how vital or impaired, whether we flourish and continue to grow, or whether we wither away. Yes, we are now age empowered.

But we're also challenged. Now accountable for our own aging experience, we're challenged to become aware of what it takes to age successfully and to incorporate this into our lives, because the MacArthur Study, in addition to showing us that more was possible, tells us that it's never too late to make a difference, to grow, to maintain what function we have now, or, at the very least, to change the slope of our decline. Luckily, the study also tells us what it takes to travel what I call this "high road to aging," to age more successfully.

The big three: a winning combination

Those who age successfully have three characteristics in common—characteristics that, in fact, define the term *successful aging*—as illustrated in figure 3.

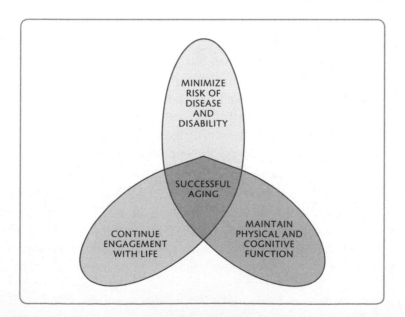

Those who age in a better way **maintain their physical and cognitive function**. Basically they *refuse to rust out*, challenging themselves physically and intellectually as a matter of lifestyle. Rather than buy into the stereotype of aging as decline, our successful agers believe that by using their faculties, whether physical or intellectual, they can at least maintain, and possibly expand, these abilities.

These aging gurus **minimize their risk of disease and disability**. They *refuse to be victims*, making great efforts to identify their risks for impairment, loss of independence, and even death and then doing all they can to *lower those risks*. Reading, researching, and working with their physicians, they become educated seekers of a lifestyle consistent with the MacArthur findings.

Lastly, and probably the most surprising finding, was that our successful agers **stayed engaged**, *refusing to be placed in the bleachers of life*, marginalized by a society that means well but still believes that "pasturizing" our older adults (like we do horses) is a good thing, a humane and caring thing. The MacArthur research shouted out to the world that older adults must *resist the isolation that is a destructive companion of growing old by remaining engaged*, defined as having a support network of friends (and family) and having *meaning and purpose in life*. When I speak on this topic, I think about our ancestors and I routinely add *being part of a community* as an essential component of being engaged in life.

A growing consensus

These findings were not that surprising. We only have to look back at our roots as a species, or even to our own lives when we were most healthy and fulfilled, to recognize these common characteristics. This has been reinforced by the recent discovery of "Blue Zones," five locations in the world where populations live significantly longer and with less disease than the rest of the world. Dan Buettner, in his November 2005 *National Geographic* article, "Secrets of Longevity," and in his book *The Blue Zones*,[4] discussed areas of the world where extreme longevity is much more common than other societies, including areas of Okinawa, Sardinia, Costa Rica, and Greece. Comparing the MacArthur Study findings, the Blue Zone characteristics, and the traits of our hunter-gatherer ancestors, we see surprising commonality. We are forced to consider that it is not serendipity that our recent research findings on successful aging are remarkably similar to the common traits of Blue Zone longevity populations, which in turn parallel characteristics of our hunter-gatherer ancestors. Might these common traits be our core needs for health and successful aging? Might these characteristics be somehow absolutes for us as humans? Authentic needs?

The following lists compare the lifestyles of our hunter-gatherer ancestors, the MacArthur Study recommendations, and Buettner's description of characteristics of Blue Zone inhabitants:

Hunter-gatherer characteristics
- highly physical
- strong social connection
- strong sense of place/purpose
- diet based on plants, fruits, nuts, fish, occasional meat/limited overall calories/obesity rare
- little chronic stress

MacArthur Study characteristics for successful aging
- physical and mental activity
- social connection
- purpose
- control of risks

Blue Zone characteristics[5]
- importance of family
- no smoking
- plant-based diet/frequent legumes
- constant moderate physical activity
- social engagement
- low chronic stress

This comparison demonstrates the enormous importance of the MacArthur Study. For the first time on a large scale, we understood aging as a multifactorial process that is largely under our control. It's not that we could substantially change the maximum lifespan of humans (that is basically determined by our uniquely human DNA), but we could influence *how* we aged, how long we remain vital, independent, and being all we can be. With this knowledge as a springboard, aging research exploded, driven by changed expectations, demographics, and, for many of the studies, the shock value of the outcomes. New findings began to come at us rapid-fire, and it was all good news.

We've learned that our brains are not the static organs we've been taught they were but instead are dynamic and alterable, with a robust potential for rewiring, growth, and healing. We are, in fact, the architects of our brains. We've learned that physical exercise is beneficial way beyond our muscles, heart, and lungs. Movement, it turns out, is critical to the functioning of all of our body's systems. For instance, movement stimulates production of what my friend Dr. David Gobble calls Miracle-Gro for our brain—BDNF, brain-derived neurotrophic factor—as well as other neurotransmitters that positively affect our mood, sleep, and outlook and significantly reduce the risk of many types of cancer. We've learned that social connection with other humans, and to some extent with animals, has a positive effect on our immune system and offers protection against heart disease, stroke, cancer, dementia, and depression. We've learned the devastating effects of the stress generated by a way of life we now consider normal but which is dramatically different from what we need in order to be healthy; the effects of this "normal" lifestyle are far more destructive than we previously thought. And we've learned that the interaction of the multiple lifestyle factors—the physical, mental, social, and spiritual—is complex, a positive health multiplier, and absolutely necessary for our health and successful aging.

The symphony of health

No longer can we fool ourselves into thinking we are healthy and doing what we need to do to age well when, in reality, we are merely going through the motions. Spending twenty minutes on an exercise bicycle (while reading a magazine) followed by overeating at our next meal; sitting and staring at a television screen for hours; regularly using drive-throughs, escalators, elevators; having others do all our physical work; eating one meal a day in order to lose weight; convincing ourselves that we are engaged in life because we multitask, cram more and more into a day, are so busy that we're always thinking of the next task, and have little time for small talk; "knowing" more because we have more answers with the help of our smartphones or the Internet; having 342 "friends" whom we never look in the eye, or touch, or cry with when they experience a loss; recycling yet driving a large SUV and frequently leaving the lights in our homes on; defining our purpose in terms of what we want rather than what we need—all these "normal" behaviors, I believe, do not meet, and in many cases are inconsistent with, the basic needs for our health handed down from our ancestors and encoded in our DNA.

I believe we must think of our health, our state of well-being, as a symphony, a thing of beauty. We are the maestro; our bodies, the orchestra; our health and aging, the music. If we are to create our own well-being—i.e., to meet all of the core requirements of authentic health—then we must be the conductor of our complex, highly integrated bodies.

The maestro must conduct in such a way that both the subtle and robust qualities of brass, percussion, strings, and woodwinds can contribute to the symphony, yet he cannot allow errant notes to mar the integrity of the piece. He must make space for all instruments to express and enhance the others, listening and staying alert to how all are blending, knowing when one needs emphasis.

As conductors of our lives, we must listen and attend to our physical, intellectual, social, and spiritual selves; we must live a life that allows coordinated expression of all we are, yet we must ensure that all its parts are in tune. We must be ever vigilant for the cacophony of self-induced stress or the overexpression of one component at the expense of the others. When we do this, and all components of the magnificent organism that is us are blended in symphonic harmony, there is an "Ode to Joy": health, vitality, and a life enriched. We age in an authentic and noble way. We are the maestro. We create a masterpiece.

My good friend Maestro David Dworkin tells me that, with each piece, the conductor has a responsibility to bring the very best of himself to the effort: energy, experience, creativity, spirituality; that each time the baton comes down, he is bringing the music alive as if it were being played for the first time. Perhaps this is why symphony conductors typically live long and robust lives and why we, as conductors of our lives, have the power to make our lives so much more.

Maestro Dworkin's own life defies traditional belief. Nearly eighty, his physical robustness rivals athletes decades younger. His intellectual curiosity and love of learning and creating are infectious. He thrives on the audiences he travels great distances to see, and to whom he offers Conductorcise®, a creation of his own that uses music to stimulate the conductor in all of us and to promote symphonies of physical, intellectual, social, and spiritual health in his audience. His passion for music and the effects it can have on humans at all stages of life is unequivocally spiritual. I believe that my friend will enrich those privileged to know him for many years to come.

Yet you need not be a maestro. My good friend Al from Pennsylvania, nearly seventy, lives a life filled with the essential characteristics of successful aging. Daily he is at the Y for a physical workout and, even more importantly, to meet with lifelong friends. He lives on a large estate but takes great pleasure in doing most of the work to maintain it. It is labor of love. He still is actively engaged in a family business started by his father, another labor of love. Surrounded by family and the rich heritage of the area he grew up in, Al is an active, connected, contented, and fulfilled man. He, too, will grace our lives for many years to come.

Remember the three key characteristics that define successful aging: low risk of disease and disease-related disability, high mental and physical function, and active engagement with life. When we commit to having these as the defining characteristics of our lifestyle, we are moving toward a better aging experience. And when we fully acknowledge that as humans we have absolute requirements in order to be truly healthy—requirements handed down from our ancestors, requirements not determined by the latest health fad but by *human experience over eons*—then now, now we have a solid road map to authentic health and successful aging. This does not mean I advocate regression to our ancestors' hunter-gatherer culture, only that we at last recognize that our basic needs for health are written in our DNA, not in the latest health advertisement, and that we find a way to acknowledge these needs in creative ways and meet them even in a culture our ancestors could never have imagined.

In the Ten Tips to Achieve Authentic Health and Successful Aging in part II of this book, I offer some recommendations that can lead to a lifestyle rich in these three basic characteristics and that will help you achieve your own version of compression—squeezing the most out of your life.

~

It is the choices we make every day that will determine whether we live the last decades of our lives slowly deteriorating, impaired and isolated, or continuing to grow, accommodating life's curveballs, staying vital and flourishing. How much we move, learn, connect with others, seek meaning, avoid creating stress, eat well—these are the decisions that determine how we will age. Making these choices not as single decisions but as a part of a commitment to a lifestyle that acknowledges our inherited human needs—this will make the difference in our lives. Such a commitment will lead us on a journey to becoming truly healthy, with a health acknowledging requirements deeply rooted in who we are as humans, wired into our very DNA, established by thousands of generations of our ancestors, and therefore authentically human. And that same journey will lead us to an aging experience filled with wonder, growth, and satisfaction.

This all makes sense, but we have to ask—is such a commitment possible?

CHAPTER 3

CAN WE CHANGE?

It is not the strongest of the species that survives, nor the
most intelligent. It is the one most adaptable to change.

—CHARLES DARWIN

I must be willing to give up what I am
in order to become what I will be.

—ALBERT EINSTEIN

See everything. Overlook a great deal. Improve a little.

—POPE JOHN XXII

This chapter is going to change everything for you. Nearly forty years of working with people to change their lives has brought me to a place where I've learned some stuff. I know that most people, particularly Americans, approach change in a way that is doomed from the beginning. It doesn't have to be that way. We can easily change the way we change. Really, we can. You can.

Life = change

The Masai people of East Africa have a saying: "Life is change." And indeed it is. Change is occurring all around us, every day, a virtual parade of transformation and alteration. We categorize it according to our personal and societal values as loss, gain, regression, renewal, growth, or decline, but no matter how we choose to classify it, it is change, and it comes with having a pulse.

We often use barometers to gauge change: clock time, birthdays, calendars, holidays, seasons, years, anniversaries, rites of passage, births, deaths. When the passage of time is subtle, like aging, we can easily fail to notice it and the change that comes with it. I have a friend who never had children, and he told me that decades passed in what seemed to be the blink of an eye, decades that parents could gauge by their children's birthdays, growth, progression in school, graduation, and marriage. If you take a mindful look, you can't help acknowledging the non-permanence around us. The faces looking back at us in the mirror are daily reminders of it. Our skin, hair, hands all are historical accounts of time passing. Even stones change. Mountains erode. Our oceans are rising, and we are all moving toward an inevitable return to the basic elements—carbon, nitrogen, oxygen, and a mix of others— that make up our bodies.

Yet, despite this universal awareness that all things change, we resist it. We set up our lives as if we believed that if we do it right, things won't change, or at least they won't get worse. We throw up virtual walls around our lives and then are surprised when the Trojan horse of sickness, or failure, or loss happens. We beat our breasts and wonder, Why me? Or, What did I do or not do that caused this change? How could this happen? Of course, change we consider good we readily accept as the fruit of our labor, or good luck. The bad, however, we psychologically resist as unwelcome and unanticipated. We spend large portions of our lives worrying about such bad change. We acquire things, relationships, status, and then fight to keep them as they are, in near-constant dread of their loss or change. Our Buddhist friends tell us that this, in fact, is the cause of most suffering in the world, our attachment to non-permanent things. Essentially, fearing that things that are fated to change actually *will* change. It is fruitless. And it is tragic.

Why do we do this? Why do we accept change on an intellectual level and resist it on a gut level? Perhaps it begins with our very existence.

We all know we will die, yet, for most of our lives, we have a feeling that somehow we will get out of this world alive. We have myths and deep faith that even if we do die, we will survive, basically as we are now, beyond death. Even without any proof whatsoever, most of us believe strongly in an afterlife.

Change inherently involves moving from what is known to what is unknown. The unknown is daunting. Contained in the unknown is a fear that under the new conditions we may fail or even not survive. I have a friend, Tom, who was a POW in Vietnam for seven years. Even under the worst of circumstances and even though he had constant hope of rescue or the end of the war, he became apprehensive when his captors moved him. Was this the end? Were the new conditions going to be worse than what he had now? We humans are highly adaptive and, indeed, that characteristic is a key to the survival and dominance of our species. Yet, despite a lifetime of successful adaptation, each one of us has a fear that the next challenge might finish us. Our bosses might find out that we're not as good as they think we are. We may not make friends in the new neighborhood we're moving to. Will I have friends when I get old? Will I have enough money after I retire? Will I die alone?

The adaptations we make to each situation we're in, over time, become comfortable. Not always in the literal sense, for there may be parts of our lives that are less than ideal. Yet, we feel secure in that we know we can manage our current life situation. Most of the time, we fully realize that "things could be worse." Additionally, ritual is comforting. Even if we are bored out of our minds, ritual can bring us an inner peace that comes with predictability. Likewise, ritual can help us "get our hands around" the change that is inevitable—births, marriages, death, and the other rites of living.

Ritual seems to appeal to us just as it did to our ancestors. And perhaps, on a very basic level, our uneasy relationship with change is a birthright handed down to us from those same ancestors, who saw so little change in their lifetimes, who valued ritual, and whose very survival was constantly threatened by any change. Change often meant threat, and with threat came fear and stress.

There are many who've excelled at aging, who understand this and have minimized change-induced stress in their lives. The New England Centenarian Study is a longitudinal study of a hundred-plus-year-old population. These very old adults share a common characteristic, which Dr. Thomas Perls, the lead investigator believes is a key element in their successful longevity formula.[1] These people know that the future holds change and adversity; after all, they know they are going to die soon. Yet they remain optimistic that whatever awaits them around the next turn in their lives, they will handle it, as they have everything else in their century-plus-long lives. Or they won't. In either case, they choose not to worry about it. They choose to live in the moment and enjoy what is now. They refuse to slide into fear, and the darkness that comes with it. And so they are open to whatever changes await them. This approach closely resembles the surrender that Buddhists advocate as a way to deal with stress, fear, and change. Not the "giving up" type of surrender, but the "I accept what is and will deal with it" surrender.

We are change veterans

The irony is that we are change survivors. In fact, we have weathered more change than any generation before us. We began the twentieth century with no airplanes, no antibiotics, only a handful of automobiles, and essentially no paved roads. Very few households had bathtubs. There were more people in Iowa than California. Even as late as forty years ago, there were no small computers, cell phones, or Internet. Yes, we're survivors. Change is indeed an ever-growing part of our lives.

And there is more irony. Despite a built-in skepticism about the change that happens *to* us, we spend a good part of lives trying to make selected change in our lives: making New Year's resolutions, trying to lose weight, quit smoking, get in better shape. This is self-imposed change, change over which we feel we have some control. This kind is perfectly acceptable to us. But frankly, we suck at it.

You know it's true. Over the course of the last year, how many times have you resolved to make substantial changes in your life? How many of those changes, if any, have you made? From the New Year's resolutions to the diets, we are terminally optimistic that we have the power to change. Please don't misunderstand. I believe we do indeed have the ability to make changes in our lives. During the course of our lives, we make many significant changes. But for most of us, those successful changes represent only a small percentage of our attempts. Some of us learn over time to accept ourselves as we are, warts and all, rather than continue to ride the roller coaster of motivation, resolution, failure, and guilt over and over again. But these people are in the minority, and nearly nonexistent among the young.

Those of us in the business of assisting people in making changes in their lives know that for change, as for so many things, there is a season. James O. Prochaska, a professor of psychology and director of the Cancer Prevention Research Center at the University of Rhode Island, developed a model for lifestyle change that assesses a person's readiness for change; for Prochaska, making this determination is the first step in any attempt to assist them in making changes.[2] Called the Transtheoretical Model of Behavior Change, this model is used by professionals like trainers, therapists, and life coaches to guide their clients through behavior change. It not only identifies six distinct stages of an individual's path to behavior change but also provides strategies for guiding people through each stage, with the ultimate goal of actual change.

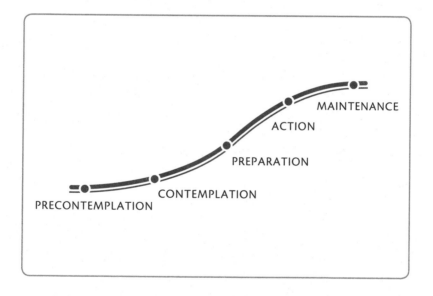

When people are felt to be in the first stage, the *precontemplative stage*, they are not thinking about making changes. In the second stage, the *contemplative stage*, they are aware of the potential benefits of change but still have enough reasons for not changing to prevent them from acting. In the next stage, the *preparation stage*, they have made up their minds to attempt to change, see the value, and begin to put their toes in the water toward the new behavior. In the *action stage*, our travelers on this change journey are "off to the races" with high hopes, motivation, and lots of ideas on how to modify their behavior in the direction of the goal. Once they've made the change and have been able to sustain the new behavior, they're in the *maintenance stage* and working to prevent relapse into old behaviors. And last comes the *termination stage* (not sure about whether that's the best term), which means that our evolving humans have reached a point where there is no temptation to return to the old behavior. The new behavior is the new normal.

This model provides some clarity in what is otherwise a free-for-all world of behavior modification. It guides the lifestyle coach or consultant, since the proper approach depends on the stage. For instance, it is fruitless to try to facilitate change in someone who is precontemplative and therefore not interested in changing. Ask any wife who had aspirations of changing her husband's behavior after they were married. Providing some basic information and backing out of the room is the recommended approach to stimulate change—an approach that allows us to concentrate on those people who are ready, thereby ensuring "more bang for the buck" from our efforts.

Of course, the Transtheoretical Model of Behavior Change is for those facilitating change in others. For ourselves, it pretty much comes down to winging it, and the results reflect this come-as-you-are, wishful-thinking approach to our own change. Having heard now what's necessary to age successfully, most of us realize we need to make some changes. So how can we do that when we are historically so bad at it?

Why we suck at change

In his intriguing book, *One Small Step Can Change Your Life*, Dr. Robert Maurer has succeeded in radically altering our views of what it takes for successful behavior change.[3] He roots our colossally consistent failure to effect change in our lives to two basic facts. First, we are wired to fear and resist large change, and second, our culture values only large change. And therein lies the dilemma. Two conditions that battle constantly and that essentially guarantee the failure of our efforts to make positive changes in our lives—two truths looking very meek alone, but that are powerful when pitted together. There is hope, however. Although one of these conditions is not alterable, the other is, and it is there that our hopes for successful behavior change lie.

Let's first address the part that we can't do too much about: the fact that we are wired to resist change.

Fear runs deep

Whatever the reason for our straight-arming of change that threatens our status quo, fear is a major player. It is a powerful inherited force in humans, as it was an absolutely necessary survival skill for our ancestors. Observations of current hunter-gatherer cultures indicate that fear, for them, seems limited to situations where there is a direct and immediate threat that demands just as immediate a response, such as during the hunting of large animals or during the response to a weather threat.

In today's hectic and competitive world, one that our ancestors could never have dreamed of, fear is self-inflicted and chronic, the by-product of our mind running rampant, chattering and creating virtual fearful situations that provoke a response, but not one that makes the fear go away. Fear of failure, injury, sickness, loss, humiliation, pain, peace, or loss of status has replaced, for the most part, the fear associated with a lion's attack. For most of us, our minds fail to keep us in the present moment, where there is rarely anything happening that generates fear. This failure to remain in the present moment, accepting this moment for what it is, without criticism or lament, realizing full well it will soon change as all things do; this failure, is a source of much of our fear as well as of its constant companion, stress (see Tip Eight).

My spiritual advisor, Yoda, the ancient Jedi master from George Lucas's *Star Wars* (whose teachings are those of famed spiritual teacher Joseph Campbell), tells us, "Fear is the path to the dark side," and he is correct. Fear cripples us and prevents us from accepting the reality of the present. Fear tortures us with negative possibilities and leaves us in a dark place indeed. Fear paralyzes us from making decisions or changes that can help us grow. Fear of change, or all the reasons for fear of change, can hold us captive, bound by invisible bonds of our own making. This fear, as we will discuss in part II, is a powerful destructive force when it comes to health and successful aging. It was protective in the simpler world of our ancestors, when it geared them up for a challenge and then dissipated when the challenge was over. But in our world, with chronic self-induced stress, which is a form of fear, it is not only not protective; it is deadly.

Fear of change is firmly rooted in our brain and isn't likely to disappear in the near future. We have a three-part brain. The most basic part we share with lower life forms and is called our "reptilian brain." The most sophisticated part distinguishes us from all other species and is called the "cerebral cortex" or "neocortex." It is here that all very high-order functions exist, and it's because of this that you are reading this at all. The middle brain, called the "midbrain" (or "paleomammalian brain"), we share with other mammals. This is control central for temperature regulation, emotion, and the famous fight-or-flight mechanism. So, when our ancestors came up over a hill and confronted a lion, this area of the brain, specifically the amygdala, jumped into action and released neurotransmitters that revved up our bodies to either *fight* the lion (a questionable decision) or run like hell—take to *flight* from the beast. The amygdala is fear central. When it fires, everything we need to fight or run is activated—and activated big-time. All body functions that aren't needed to deal with the situation are slowed down, ignored, or inactivated. It is efficient. It is effective. It is perfect.

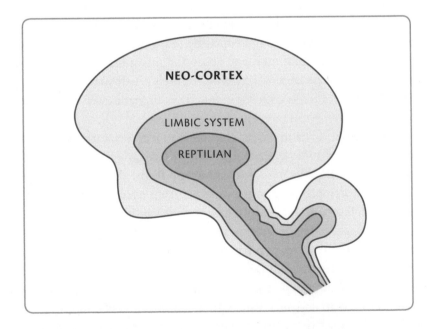

Compared to today, not too much happened in our ancestors' world, and when it did, there was a good chance that survival itself was at stake.

So when change came, it grabbed our ancestors' attention. In fact, it more often than not caused them to fear the change. So the amygdala was called into action and, as programmed, revved up all the fight-or-flight systems and shut down other bodily functions, like digestion, urination, and thinking. After all, confronting a lion was not a good time to rid ourselves of waste, or think about how you're going to get away. It was all automatic. Threat (change) caused fear, and fear caused everything to shut down except what was needed to fight or run. It's that simple, and this response remains with us today. So what about the part we *can* do something about?

"No fear"—the path to change

Change, Dr. Maurer tells us, especially the big bites of change we all characteristically take on, triggers this same instinctual fear. We are wired that way. It may be masked as anxiety, uncertainty, or a zealot-like attempt to change, but it is, in the end, fear. So if we hit our brains with a New Year's resolution to lose twenty-five pounds, or to be nicer to our spouse, or to learn Italian, we are causing our amygdala to act as if a lion were in our house. Just when we need purposeful thinking, creativity, a rational reason why we should change, and a plan for targeted, purposeful action, our brains essentially shut down because of fear. It is fear that causes us to fail, not succeed. Fear that grabs us precisely when we need a clear mind to develop a plan to change, when we need a reason to change, and when we need higher purpose to suppress our more basic instincts. This fear makes us fearful idiots precisely when we need all of our higher faculties to chart a course to constructive change.

Dr. Maurer is a clinical psychologist, and his answer to this dilemma is to change how we approach change, taking on smaller bites instead of our usual big bites. He advocates *kaizen*, the Japanese technique for making change, whether in our personal lives or in business. Kaizen is about small changes, easily achievable goals that are so small they do not trigger the amygdala to go into alert mode. Goals that might seem ridiculous by our current standards can slip by the amygdala—i.e., not generate fear, or modern-day stress—and therefore leave our needed faculties intact to bring the change to reality.

Katie Sloan is the chief operating officer, senior vice president, and executive director of the International Association of Homes and Services for the Aging (IAHSA) and a colleague of mine. In a speech she gave at Masterpiece Living's annual meeting, called "The Lyceum," in 2011, she gave me the clearest picture of the value of this small-step approach to change. She said that if we are walking and make no change whatsoever, we will end up at destination A. If we change our direction only slightly, by just two or three degrees, in time we will end up at destination B, *a long way from destination A!* With just small changes, persistence, and patience, we can make huge changes in our lives.

The way we approach change in our "take no prisoners" society, however, is not as Katie describes it. We do it by innovation, described by Maurer as "a drastic process of change," which ideally "occurs in a very short period of time, yielding a dramatic turnaround." Sound familiar? Sound like every New Year's resolution you ever made? Sound like the typical American approach to weight loss? Don't think I'm against innovation. Who could be? However, when it is the standard for behavior change, it is usually too ambitious, and at high risk of failure. Why? You got it: It generates fear, maybe of failure, or loss of the familiar, whatever, but fear that shuts down the higher-level cortical functions we need to succeed. As Dr. Maurer tells us, "Change is frightening. . . . This fear of change is rooted in the brain's physiology, and when fear takes hold, it can prevent creativity, change, and success."

John Wooden, one of most successful coaches in college basketball, knew how to make positive change happen. "Don't look for the big, quick improvement. Seek the small improvement one day at a time. That's the only way it happens—and when it happens, it lasts."[4] That's kaizen.

Kaizen is about small steps. It's about *asking ourselves small questions*: "What is the simplest thing I can do to begin moving?" "What can I do in five minutes each day to become more positive?" Small questions allow us to begin thinking about a plan for change without triggering the amygdala and setting up roadblocks to success.

Kaizen is about *mind sculpture*, a technique described by Ian Robertson in his book by the same title.[5] With mind sculpture, we imagine ourselves performing the activity that we want to do, and use our senses to do the imagining: feeling the muscles move, smelling the associated smells, hearing the sounds, seeing ourselves performing the act, not as a viewer would view us, but what we would see as we actually performed it.

Maurer tells us that "within minutes of 'practicing' a task mentally, using all your senses, the brain's chemistry begins to change. It rewires its cells and the connections between the cells to create complex motor or verbal skills." Brain-imaging capabilities have allowed us to "see" this brain activity going on as if the action were really happening. We "fool" our brains into making connections without the fear normally associated with new tasks or behaviors. We rewire our brains so that the desired behavior happens easily, without the amygdala sounding the alarm, without stress or fear impeding our progress toward a new, more positive behavior. Even just a few seconds or minutes each day can build these new brain connections and allow us to actually perform the new behavior without the usual roadblocks.

Kaizen is about *taking small steps*. Having asked ourselves small questions, decided what small action we might do to change our lives, and used mind sculpture to practice that action and begin to make brain connections that will make it easy to perform, we now take small steps toward our goal. We're talking *ridiculously* small steps by current standards. Like learning one word of a new language a day, or walking ten more steps each day, or thinking one nice thing about someone. These small steps will not trigger the brain's survival/fear/change response. The amygdala will remain quiet. We will feel positive about what we've done, but more importantly, about our ability to change. And we'll be on our way toward whatever we want to accomplish.

Kaizen is about *solving small problems*. True, if our doctor tells us we must lose fifty pounds, that's not a small problem. But asking ourselves small questions, seeing ourselves find the answer to those questions, and taking small steps, like beginning to stand during TV commercials, or spitting out the first bite of a candy bar—those are small changes, baby steps on a journey that will become easier as we accomplish small tasks without fear, without failure. And even when we do "fail," we have only to take a small step backward to get on track. And as we collect more and more successes, no matter how small, we make huge gains in confidence, and, by adding small increments of change, ultimately eat the elephant, one small bite at a time.

Can we change?

Of course we can. We must, if we are to navigate through a lifetime where the rate of change is ever rising, where whether we prosper, stay healthy, or age successfully is all dependent on our ability to make corrections to, refine, and otherwise modify our behavior. We must.

Dr. Maurer tells us, "Instead of aggressively forcing yourself into a boot-camp mentality about change, give your mind permission to make the leaps on its own schedule, in its own time."[6]

So out with the "just do it" New Year's resolution, the never-again, seesaw, guilt-ridden approach to bettering ourselves. As some ask, "How's that working for you?" If it has, terrific; however, you are in the minority. As for us mere mortals, a more modest approach will serve us well. So, when you're considering making some changes in your life, consider the kaizen way:

- Identify specifically *why* you want to change.
- Then zero in on *what* you want to change.
- Ask yourself, "What's the smallest thing I can do to begin this change?"
- Make that small thing—and *not* the ultimate change—your goal.
- Imagine yourself doing that thing.
- When you achieve the small goal, add the next smallest thing you can do.
- If you fail to achieve a goal, just step back to the last achieved goal and add a smaller, more achievable goal to that.
- Keep adding very small increments to your progress. It doesn't matter how long it takes. You are changing, and moving toward your ultimate goal.

And remember, the journey is as important as the destination.

CHAPTER 4

YOUR PERSONAL LIFESTYLE INVENTORY

*If we want to grow, we must change. If we are to
going to change, we must make changes.*

It's the moment of, and for, truth. We've talked about our ancestors and how the way they lived over eons determined what we as their descendants need to be healthy and to age well. We've learned that their lifestyle is, in fact, a guide to our most basic needs, our authentic human needs as humans. We've noted that how we live today is radically different from how our ancestors lived, and that therefore we are a species with Stone Age needs in a microchip world, and we've seen how we are paying the price. Recent research has revealed what it takes to be truly healthy and age well, and those revelations look remarkably like those authentic human needs laid down by our ancestors. We know we can't go back in time, but we can—by knowing what it takes to become authentically healthy and to age successfully—begin to bring these things back into our lives.

So now is your moment. Your moment to honestly assess your current lifestyle. Your moment to find out how far you may have wandered from your basic human needs for health. Your moment to find out just where you are at risk for disease or accelerated decline. This can be scary, I know—I've done it myself. But not to worry. These are easy questions to answer. The hard part is answering them truthfully. Your answers will help guide you to the best recommendations for aging in a better way, a more enjoyable way, a more successful way. There are no right answers, only *your* answers. When you have completed the Personal Lifestyle Inventory, consult the feedback section immediately following. This feedback will help you interpret your score and, most importantly, provide you guidance on which of the Ten Tips in part II of this book are particularly important to you.

The Ten Tips offer practical, easy-to-do things you can use to get back on track: things you can do to begin to navigate your way through all the health and aging advice that's out there, telling you to do this and that, some impossible, some contradictory, some just plain crazy. The Ten Tips are the result of my decades of experience in taking personal histories to uncover disease and its causes as well as to determine the best plan of action. In Masterpiece Living communities, we use similar questions in order to determine an individual's risk to their health and independence. I'm sure you, too, will find them to be "just what the doctor ordered."

As you complete this evaluation and find out what you need to do to get started down the road to authentic health and successful aging, it will be as if your ancestors are whispering in your ear, giving you a sense of true north when it comes to living a healthy life. All you need to do is listen and learn. Thousands living in Masterpiece Living communities have done it. So can you.

1. How much total time do you spend moving your body during an average day (walking, exercising, doing physical work)?

   a) Less than one hour b) Between one and two hours c) Over two hours

2. How many people did you share a face-to-face conversation with today that lasted longer than two minutes?

   a) None b) One or two c) Three or more

3. How many days last week did you learn something new or do something you've never done before?

   a) None b) One or two c) Three or more

4. Are you proud of your answer when someone asks how you spend your day?

   a) Not proud b) A little proud c) Very proud

5. How many servings of fruits, vegetables, or nuts do you eat *most* days?

   a) Less than two b) Between two and four c) Five or more

6. What is the difference between your current weight and what you weighed at age eighteen?

   a) Twenty pounds or more b) Between ten and twenty pounds
   c) Ten pounds or less

7. How many times today did you feel in a rush?

   a) Three or more b) One or two c) None

8. How much do you worry?

   a) A lot b) Some, but it's under control
   c) Very little. It's a waste of time.

9. How often are you thinking about things other than what you're currently doing?

   a) Often b) Sometimes c) Hardly ever

10. Are you pleased with the quality of your sleep?

    a) Not at all b) Somewhat pleased c) Very pleased

11. How many times did you laugh today (not just smile, but laugh for longer than two seconds)?

    a) None b) Once c) Twice or more

12. How long has it been since you last interacted with a child?

    a) Months or years b) Weeks c) Days

Your Personal Inventory Score and Feedback

1. **How much total time do you spend moving your body during an average day (walking, exercising, doing physical work)?**

   a) Less than one hour   **(5 points)**

   You are classified as sedentary or nearly so. Such little physical movement is dramatically different from how we evolved as humans and potentially puts you at high risk for multiple diseases and limitations, including heart disease, stroke, diabetes, some cancers, osteoporosis, and even early dementia. Please consult Tips One and Two. Tip Three also contains information regarding physical activity and brain health that you will find helpful. Please also revisit chapter 3, to establish realistic goals for change. I know you can lower your risks and improve your life. Live well!

b) Between one and two hours   (7 points)

You are potentially at some risk for multiple diseases and limitations, including heart disease, stroke, diabetes, some cancers, osteoporosis, and even dementia. Please consult Tips One, Two, and Three. Please also revisit chapter 3 to establish realistic goals for change. You can build on your current activity level to reduce your risks even further. Live well!

c) Over two hours   (10 points)

Congratulations! You are better than most of your peers with your current level of physical activity. This dramatically reduces your risk of heart disease, stroke, diabetes, some cancers, osteoporosis, and even dementia. I encourage you to continue to build on this level of activity to further reduce your risks and improve your likelihood for aging more successfully. Please consult Tips One, Two, and Three for encouragement and some ideas for enhancing your physical self. Keep up the good work. Live well!

My Score (question 1)_____

2. **How many people did you share a face-to-face conversation with today that lasted longer than two minutes?**

   ### a) None   (3 points)

   If this is a usual day for you, then you're effectively living a life of relative isolation. You are not meeting your inherited need for social interaction and engagement, even though this is important to authentic health and successful aging. You are potentially at high risk for a number of serious conditions, including heart disease, cancer, depression, and dementia. There is a high probability your immune system is adversely affected by this isolation. Please consult Tip Four to begin lowering your risk. Revisit chapter 3 for additional guidance on setting expectations. You may feel some initial discomfort, but you can become more socially engaged, and you'll feel better than you ever expected. Be well!

b) One or two   (7 points)

If this is a usual day, you are like most of your peers in that you are living a life with limited social engagement. We have an inherited need as humans for regular social interaction; authentic health and successful aging both depend on it. With limited social engagement, you are potentially at risk for heart disease, cancer, depression, dementia, and a weakened immune system. To build on your current level of social interaction, please consult Tip Four. Revisit chapter 3 for guidance on setting expectations. I'm sure you will be successful, and that the quality of your life will significantly improve. Be well and engaged!

c) Three or more   (10 points)

Congratulations! If this is a usual day, then it is most likely you are socially well engaged, which is a critical component of being authentically healthy and aging successfully. You probably have a significantly lower risk of heart disease, cancer, depression, and dementia. Your immune system is also more likely to be functioning at high effectiveness. To build on your commendable current level, please consult Tip Four, and remember the guidance in chapter 3 as you become even more socially engaged. Keep up the great work! What you are doing will pay off in the quality of your life.

My Score (question 2)_____

My Cumulative Score (questions 1–2) _____

3. **How many days last week did you learn something new or do something you've never done before?**

a) None   (3 points)

Our new knowledge of how the brain works reveals that we are the architects of our brain. We can stimulate growth of new connections that can help us stay sharp and delay (and maybe prevent) the onset of dementia. This happens when we *learn and do new things.* You are potentially at risk for less-than-ideal brain aging and even early-onset dementia. See Tip Three for guidance on starting a brain-fitness lifestyle. If you consult chapter 3, you will see that it is not difficult and even fun. Anyone can do it and, of course, *you* can do it. Be prepared for an enjoyable and empowering journey once you take the first small steps.

b) One or two   (7 points)

Every time you learn and do new things, you are wiring your brain in a new way, making new connections. This is very healthy for the brain, keeping it vital and responsive. Your willingness to learn and do new things potentially lowers your risk for the onset of the symptoms of dementia, and quite possibly will influence whether you'll ever get symptoms at all. Consult Tip Three for ways to build on your current level of brain fitness. Remember the advice in chapter 3 on taking small steps toward healthy change and successful aging of the brain. Enjoy your new journey of discovery and brain fitness.

c) Three or more   (8 points)

Congratulations! You are a brain-fitness gold medalist. Your willingness to try new things is going to serve you, and your brain, very well. You are the architect of your brain and you are enhancing and rewiring it continuously. This is associated with positive effects on your risk for the development of the symptoms of dementia. We may soon discover it can prevent dementia altogether. In the meantime, keep up your inspiring approach to life and brain health and continue putting yourself out there and trying new things. Consult Tip Three and chapter 3 for additional guidance. Enjoy your journey!

My Score (question 3) _____

My Cumulative Score (questions 1–3) _____

4. **Are you proud of your answer when someone asks how you spend your day?**

a) Not proud   (3 points)

I'm sorry to hear this. We all deserve to be proud of our lives. The MacArthur Study found that having purpose in life is, in fact, one of the key characteristics of people who age successfully. Volunteerism brings more longevity, better memory, and greater overall health. Understand that you don't have to save lives to have great purpose. The important thing is that you have a meaningful reason to get out of bed in the morning. It could be a garden, or helping handicapped children, or fighting to rid the world of hunger. Oftentimes, the simplest things we do can bring purpose, yet we undervalue them and feel we have no purpose. For most people, purpose involves other living things, whether people, animals, or plants. Please consult Tip Eight for help with finding purpose. Tips Four, Seven, Nine, and Ten may also be of help. Revisit chapter 3 for guidance in setting goals. You can do this. It will make all the difference. Start today.

b) A little proud   (6 points)

This is working for you. Purpose is key for aging successfully and enhances the overall quality of life. Having something *you* consider worth getting out of bed in the morning for makes all the difference. Volunteering is associated with longevity, better memory, and overall health. It matters little what that is, but for most, it involves other living things. Consult Tip Four for more help building on the sense of purpose you currently have. Tips Seven, Nine, and Ten may also be of help. Revisiting chapter 3 can assist you in establishing realistic goals. You have a foundation, and that will help you in your desire to find even greater purpose in your life. Good luck!

c) Very proud   (8 points)

Congratulations! Being proud of how you spend your time indicates that you have purpose. Purpose is critical to successful aging. If you are still working, are you sure your purpose will be there after you stop? Most often, purpose that is resilient over a lifespan involves doing something for other living things. Consult Tip Three for some guidance on how to build on the firm foundation of purpose you currently have and to help you with establishing realistic goals for the future. Keep up the good work. You are a standout among your peers.

My Score (question 4) _____

My Cumulative Score (questions 1–4) _____

5. **How many servings of fruits, vegetables, or nuts do you eat most days?**

   a) Less than two (4 points)

   For most of the time that we humans have lived, we ate a diet of fruits, wild vegetables, nuts, fish, and small amounts of meat. Grains and meat are a relatively new addition to our diets, at least in the quantities that we eat today. Sugar, except that found naturally in these foods, was a foreign substance. It is no wonder, then, that fruits, vegetables, and nuts are so important in keeping us healthy. It's not that meats and grains are necessarily bad for us; it's just that they should be eaten in smaller quantities, as opposed to at least five, if not more, helpings of fruits, vegetables, and nuts. Simple sugars, as are found in soft drinks, candy, and pastries, should be considered *very* special treats. Our systems are not geared to handle large amounts of such sugar, and eating large amounts can result in obesity, diabetes, and increased risk of other chronic illnesses. Please consult Tips Five and Three. Most importantly, return to chapter 3 for a realistic, Aristotle-like ("All things in moderation") approach to improving your diet. Remember, diet is more about the proper fuel for our bodies than it is about weight. Eat correctly and keep moving, and weight is less likely to be a problem. Be patient. You can do this.

   b) Between two and four (6 points)

   You are doing better than most of your peers but are nevertheless falling short of what your body needs to be in optimum health, perform at its best, and be at its best weight. For most of the time we humans have been on earth, we've eaten mostly fruits, vegetables, nuts, fish, and small amounts of meat. Meats and grains are a relatively new addition to our diets, at least in the quantities we eat today. So it is understandable that our bodies require fruits, vegetables, and nuts more than anything else. So, build on the good work you're doing and make a plan to add at least two or more servings of fruits, vegetables, or nuts to your daily diet. Consult Tips Five and Three for guidance and chapter 3 for advice on making a plan to change. You're already including good foods in your diet, so take the next steps to put you over the top on a diet that will keep you healthy, performing at your best, and maintaining a weight that will reduce your risk of many serious diseases and conditions.

c) Five or more   (8 points)

Congratulations! You are eating foods that your body needs to stay healthy, to perform at its best, and to maintain a better weight. Fruits, vegetables, nuts, fish, and small amounts of meat were the primary diet of humans for most of the time we have walked the earth and are absolutely necessary for health and performance. Meat and grains in the quantities we eat them today are relatively new additions to our diets, and, although good foods, should not be the primary elements of our daily diets. Eating fruits, vegetables, and nuts in the quantities you are eating them usually results in the balanced diet we all need. So again, congratulations. Keep up the good work, and if you enjoy these foods, you probably cannot get too much of them. Well done!

My Score (question 5) _____

My Cumulative Score (questions 1–5) _____

6. What is the difference between your current weight and what you weighed at age eighteen?

(Note: This is only a rough gauge of healthy weight. For most of us over fifty years old, we were at a healthy adult weight at age eighteen. A better indicator of healthy weight is the body mass index, or BMI. You can easily calculate your BMI by using the National Heart, Lung, and Blood Institute's calculator at www.nhlbisupport. com/bmi.)

a) Twenty pounds or more   (3 points)

You are at higher risk for a number of conditions associated with being overweight or obese (see the BMI calculation). Many of these conditions are serious threats to your independence, quality of life, and, in fact, your life itself. Conditions associated with being overweight or obese include coronary heart disease, stroke, type 2 diabetes, cancer, osteoarthritis, sleep apnea, high blood pressure, and high blood fats. Please see Tip Five for guidance. It is very important that you review chapter 3 for a realistic approach to weight loss and health. Tips One and Two will also offer some sound advice. Be patient. Be realistic. Be persistent. You can do this. You will reap huge rewards with each pound lost. Go for it!

b) Between ten and twenty pounds (6 points)

Like most people, you have probably very gradually added weight over many years. You probably don't even consider yourself overweight, but the BMI calculation should be your guide. If indeed your BMI classifies you as overweight, you are at moderately higher risk for a number of potentially serious conditions: coronary heart disease, stroke, type 2 diabetes, cancer, osteoarthritis, sleep apnea, high blood pressure, high blood fats, and more. Many of these conditions can adversely affect your aging experience and even threaten your independence. Please see Tip Five for guidance. Tips One and Two may also be of some interest. It is very important that you review chapter 3 for a realistic approach to weight loss and health. Be patient. Be realistic. Be persistent. You can achieve a healthier weight and reap significant health, quality-of-life, and aging benefits.

c) Ten pounds or less (8 points)

Congratulations! Despite the decades it's been since you were eighteen years old, you have maintained an apparent healthy weight. Calculate your BMI (see above instructions) to be sure. If your BMI is in the recommended range, you are at lower risk for many serious chronic diseases, including heart disease, cancer, diabetes, and stoke. Please consult Tips Five and Three for additional dietary guidance. If indeed you decide to make a change in your lifestyle, eating habits, or weight, please return to chapter 3 for guidance. Keep up the great work!

My Score (question 6) _____

My Cumulative Score (questions 1–6) _____

7. How many times today did you feel in a rush?

a) Three or more (4 points)

You are potentially at high risk for the adverse effects of chronic stress. The list of possible stress-related diseases is extensive and includes heart disease, depression, some cancers, gastrointestinal disorders, and even dementia. Since most stress is, in fact, self-induced, you have the opportunity to lower your risks substantially. This is important not only for disease prevention but for quality of life and relationships. Please consult Tips Five and Seven for an understanding of the role of stress and for some stress-reduction recommendations. As you attempt to make changes, remember the advice from chapter 3. This is a challenge for you, but you have the potential to achieve great rewards. Good luck!

b) One or two   (6 points)

Although you are probably like most people you know when it comes to feeling rushed and stressed, that doesn't help the fact that you are potentially at some risk for the adverse effects of stress. The list of possible stress-related diseases is extensive and includes heart disease, depression, some cancers, gastrointestinal disorders, and even dementia. Since most stress is, in fact, self-induced, you have the opportunity to lower your risks substantially. This is important not only for disease prevention but for quality of life and relationships. Please consult Tips Five and Seven for an understanding of the role of stress and for some stress-reduction recommendations. As you attempt to make changes, remember the approach outlined in chapter 3.

c) None   (8 points)

Congratulations! If this represents your usual day, you are unusual compared to your peers. Chronic stress is rampant throughout our society, as we accept over-scheduling and overstimulation as a part of normal life. You realize that most stress is self-induced and is therefore something we can control through our lifestyle decisions. I'm hopeful you can continue your mindful approach to life, your realistic expectations, and your mindful use of technology. Tips Five and Seven can provide some validation of your current lifestyle. Keep up the great work!

My Score (question 7) _____

My Cumulative Score (questions 1–7) _____

8. How much do you worry?

a) A lot   (3 points)

Welcome to a very large group, yet one with high risk for a long list of stress-related disorders and associated lower quality of life. You may feel that you have reason to worry, but in truth, worry accomplishes no good, instead potentially causes much bad, and is for the most part a self-induced phenomenon. Honestly, it is. It is essential that we all learn that when confronted with a difficult situation, we fix it, walk away, or accept it. There are no other solutions. Chronic worry about situations is a major threat. Please consult Tips Five and Seven. Tips Eight, Nine, and Ten will also offer some assistance in your search for peace. Chapter 3 will guide you in your journey of change. I wish you success.

b) Some, but it's under control   (6 points)

Clearly you recognize the potential deleterious effects of worry on health and aging. It's true: none of us are free of worry, even though that freedom is possible and an important part of authentic health and successful aging. Instead of making worry a part of your life, fix the situation, walk away, or accept it. Even a little worry is potentially harmful. Don't *worry* about it. Rather, consult Tips Five and Seven for guidance. Remember the advice in chapter 3 regarding making change.

c) Very little. It's a waste of time.   (8 points)

Congratulations! I'd like to give you more points. You have broken the code for authentic health, successful aging, and a high quality of life. Fix it. Walk away. Or accept it. Those are the options. Worry is a waste of time. I applaud your lifestyle choice—for indeed, it is a choice. I hope your choice has a positive effect on those you come in contact with. It's a rare quality that we need more of. Keep up the good work!

My Score (question 8) _____

My Cumulative Score (questions 1–8) _____

9. **How often are you thinking about things other than what you're currently doing?**

a) Often   (3 points)

Of course, you are not alone, but this disease of chattering mind puts you at high risk for a long list of stress-related disorders, for lower-quality relationships, for lower quality of life, and for an absence of peace. Runaway thoughts prevent us from making good decisions and appreciating what is important in our lives. Some would call this the scourge of our age. If you were to work on any of your problem areas, I recommend you consider this one a very high priority. It's not easy. I recommend you review Tips Seven and Five. Additionally, I recommend Tips Eight, Nine, and Ten. I wish you success in this important journey.

b) Sometimes   (6 points)

You are not alone, but that will not be comforting as you struggle with this risk to the quality of your life and relationships, as well as to your health and aging. The ability to "be in the moment" is rare but comes with very high rewards. As long as we accept chattering mind as normal, we will not seek out readily available strategies to move toward a lifestyle more consistent with our origins as a species and therefore more conducive to authentic health. Tips Five and Seven can assist you in your journey toward this lifestyle. Good luck!

c) Hardly ever   (8 points)

Congratulations. You are my hero. Moreover, you are the type of person I enjoy having discussions with. You have achieved a lifestyle that is rare but that is hopefully becoming more common. Being "in the moment" allows you to have high-quality relationships and a higher quality of life and significantly lowers your risk of stress-related disorders. I applaud your accomplishment and recommend Tips Five and Seven to validate your lifestyle choice. Keep up the good work!

My Score (question 9) _____

My Cumulative Score (questions 1–9) _____

10. Are you pleased with the quality of your sleep?

a) Not at all   (3 points)

I'm sorry. This is indeed an affliction and it puts you at high risk for accidents and stress-related disorders, including depression, and lowers your overall quality of life. I highly recommend that you discuss this with your doctor to ensure there is not a medical condition causing your poor sleep. If a medical condition is not responsible, there are multiple strategies to improve sleep, including those contained in the US Department of Health and Human Services booklet *Your Guide to Healthy Sleep*. For many, stress or worry is the cause of poor sleep. For this, I recommend Tips Five, Seven, Eight, Nine, and Ten. Remember to make small changes toward your goal, and revisit chapter 3 for advice on change.

b) Somewhat pleased   (6 points)

Sleep is critical to us for optimal functioning as well as for lowering the risk for many disorders, including depression and other stress-related conditions. I recommend you review the booklet *Your Guide to Healthy Sleep* put out by the US Department of Health and Human Services. Make sure you ask your physician if you have any conditions that might interfere with your sleep. If not, it may be stress or worry that is interfering. Consult Tips Five and Seven. Also review Tips Eight, Nine, and Ten for additional guidance.

c) Very pleased   (8 points)

Congratulations! You have a gift that will serve you well, keeping you healthy and aging well, and giving you a higher quality of life and lower risk of disease. Whatever you're doing, it's working for you. Keep up the good work!

My Score (question 10) _____

My Cumulative Score (questions 1–10) _____

11. How many times did you laugh today (not just smile, but laugh for longer than two seconds)?

a) None   (3 points)

Sorry to hear that. Laughing is associated with healthier immune systems; lowered risk for many disorders, including depression; better relationships; and a higher quality of life. Even forced laughter is healthy. Beyond that, addressing worry and stress can be a significant step toward laughter and its associated benefits. Please review Tips Ten, Five, and Seven. Tip Eight can also be useful. The list of stress-related diseases is extensive and includes heart dis-ease, depression, some cancers, gastrointestinal disorders, and even dementia. Since most stress is, in fact, self-induced, you have the opportunity to lower your risks substantially. This is important not only for disease prevention but for quality of life and relationships. As you attempt to make changes, revisit chapter 3 and remember that change should be in small steps. Good luck in your journey. Even small gains will feel good.

b) Once   (6 points)

I'll take it. Even one laugh is beneficial—and the day's not over! Truly, laughter stimulates our immune system, improves our mood, and increases our quality of life. Look for more opportunities to laugh, for with laughter will come reduced risk of many conditions, including, of course, depression and, potentially, dementia. Review Tip Ten. You may also find good advice in Tips Seven, Five, and Nine. Keep laughing!

c) Twice or more   (8 points)

Congratulations! You're the kind of person I regularly seek out. Your ability to see humor and to laugh is serving you well in reducing the risk of many stress-related disorders, including depression. Your immune system is benefiting, as are your relationships and your overall quality of life. Keep laughing!

My Score (question 11) _____

My Cumulative Score (questions 1–11) _____

12. How long has it been since you last interacted with a child?

a) Months or years   (4 points)

Both you and some children are missing out. I understand how this can happen, but it need not, and the benefits to your health and aging make it even more imperative that you seek out opportunities that are not available to you now. Although we cannot point to any particular disease caused by lack of association with children, we are clear that it is a fundamental human requirement for optimum functioning. Children are the continuance of our lives—viewed on a grand scale, our lives are more relevant because of them. Whether it's about our enjoyment, purpose, or socialization, children play an essential role. It's easy to fall into a lifestyle where children are not present. It's easy to assume life is easier without children. I challenge you to interact with children; the fulfillment they bring will, I'm certain, become obvious to you. Please consult Tips Nine, Eight, and Ten. There's a new life awaiting you. Good luck on your journey.

b) Weeks   (6 points)

Indeed, it can be difficult to keep children in your life. I encourage you to continue to make the effort, for the benefits to your quality of life and risk of disease are substantial. Look ahead and plan how you will keep children, or at least younger people, in your life. Consult Tips Nine and Eight for guidance. Keep up the fun!

c) Days   (8 points)

Congratulations! I don't have to tell you how children enhance our lives. You should know, however, that intergenerational contact is associated with lowered risk of many disorders and with enhanced quality of life and better aging. Remember, kids grow up, so plan on how to keep children in your life. Keep up the good work!

My Score (question 12) _____

My Cumulative Score (questions 1–12) _____

Cumulative Score Analysis

90–100   Congratulations!

You are a lifestyle gold medalist. Your lifestyle is indeed a symphony, for you are clearly paying attention to all the dimensions that influence your health and aging: the physical, intellectual, social, and spiritual. You're managing your stress and remaining positive about the next phase of your life. I applaud your efforts but caution you to stay alert. Life has a way of surprising us with challenges that can easily knock us off track. So, take this assessment every six months and keep mindful of the basic lifestyle requirements to stay authentically healthy and age successfully. Keep up the great work!

75–89   You're on track.

And you're beating the odds right now with your current lifestyle. That's not to say you're not still at risk, but you're clearly making efforts to be healthy and age in a better way. These efforts are paying off but are still falling short of what your efforts could do. So, look at the areas where you're at risk, read the recommendations in the sections addressing those risks, and begin making small changes toward more authentic health and more successful aging. Your efforts won't be wasted; I guarantee it. Onward and upward.

60–74   There's room for improvement.

OK, so you're doing well in some areas but you're also still at risk for some bad stuff happening to you—stuff that could threaten your independence and quality of life. So let's take this as a wake-up call. Remember, it's never too late to make positive changes that can lower your risks and put you on the road to authentic health and successful aging. Don't worry about it; just find out the areas where you're at risk and read the recommendations that apply to those areas. Take small steps and *you will improve*. I guarantee it. Just be patient, be clear on what you want to achieve, and keep pressing, even when you fall short. Be in it for the long haul, because that's what you want your life to be—long, and not encumbered by impairments that come with chronic disease. You can do this. Remember, it's never too late—or too early.

Below 60   This book is a great investment!

The good news is that you're going to benefit most by reading this book. The bad news is that you're at significant risk for very bad stuff happening that can potentially threaten your independence and your quality of life. This isn't time to beat your breast or call yourself names; it's time to celebrate the fact that you've taken the first step toward authentic health and successful aging by *knowing you're at risk*. Knowing this, and knowing specifically what you're at risk for, puts you light years ahead of many of your peers. Now, knowing what to do about those risks—well, that puts you in a great place to jump ahead with your life. *The biggest danger for you is trying to do too much too soon, and losing confidence that you can make a differ-ence.* So, look at where you're at risk, review the recommendations for those areas, and review chapter 3, which helps you set realistic goals. Then begin! Be patient, be realistic, be confident you can do it, *because you can do this!* There is no specific timetable, but you must begin now if you want to reap the huge rewards that are waiting for you to claim. OK? Good. Onward and upward.

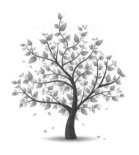

PART II

TEN TIPS TO ACHIEVE AUTHENTIC HEALTH AND SUCCESSFUL AGING

Confront the difficult while it is still easy;
accomplish the great task by a series of small acts.
—TAO TE CHING

I hope from what you wanted, you get what you need.
—JUDY COLLINS, "BORN TO THE BREED"

*I*f you have a pulse, there are risks out there, circling overhead like buzzards, waiting for a moment when you're weak, or susceptible, or less resilient. Whether it's a cold or cancer, these threats are out there, waiting to swoop in. What keeps them at bay is your resilience, resilience developed by a lifestyle that builds up your physical, mental, social, and spiritual strength and results in authentic health—*the state of genuine* *vitality consistent with our human origins and individual nature.* This is health resulting in resilience, and it is achieved by deliberate attention to not just one or two of the components that make us human but all of them. Medicine may have fractionated us into a cardiovascular system, a neurologic system, a gastrointestinal system, and more, but we are *whole integrated beings*, more than the sum of our parts. The interaction of the ten trillion cells and multiple systems and unique experiences and emotions, the smooth interaction and attention to the whole, is what keeps us alive and healthy even as we age. This smooth interaction might also be called "holistic" or "whole-person strength." As in our analogy of an exceptional symphony orchestra, each cell, each organ, each system interacts and blends with others to create one functioning organism that is, again, more than the sum of the parts.

Threats to our health and successful aging are not only always present; they are also always looking for opportunities, any sign of vulnerability in us. Are we depressed? Is the Big Uneasy—stress—compromising our immune defenses? Are we eating poorly? Have we become sedentary, or obese? Are we not getting enough sleep? Are we isolated from others? Are we negative or pessimistic? Do we have no purpose or passion about living? All of these are holes in our defenses. Our health and successful aging are a finely tuned, complicated choreography of whole-body strength: physical, mental, social, and spiritual; all necessary, like links on a chain. When we pay attention to all these, we are being true to our human roots; we are rediscovering our ancestral legacy. We are being *authentic* to the core of our human needs and not allowing ourselves to be distracted by the latest health fad or claim for miraculous transformation of our bodies and minds.

This whole-body strength is the result our lifestyle, the choices we make every day. And what is the lifestyle that can build this strength and resilience? The ten tips that make up part II of this book are a guide to building and maintaining that lifestyle, developing resilience, and keeping disease, particularly the chronic disease that saps our independence and quality of life, at bay. Buddhists use the term *spiritual warrior* to describe one who combats self-ignorance, which they believe is the source of suffering in the world. Perhaps then, by helping us overcome our own ignorance about what makes us sick and what keeps us well and resilient, the Ten Tips are a guide to becoming a warrior for your own true, authentic health and successful aging.

How to use the Ten Tips

The results and feedback of your Personal Lifestyle Inventory (which I highly recommend you take) will point you to specific areas in this section, but whether you took the inventory or not, the Ten Tips are the key to building the resilience you'll need to weather life's slings and arrows, or, if you prefer, life's curveballs.

Read all of the Ten Tips in part II. Then concentrate on those areas your inventory feedback indicated needed attention or any areas you would like to strengthen. Remember, we can have many strong links, but if there is even one weak link, we are vulnerable. At the end of each tip, you will find suggestions for converting what you have just learned into action. These Masterpiece Living Pearls are gems of advice collected from the experience of seeing thousands of older adults change their lives. These suggestions have worked for them, and will work for you.

Reread the tips as often as you like. You will take away something new each time: something that resonates more with where you are in your personal journey. You will see overlap within them. This only reinforces the fact that we are one whole being with many interdependent components. Remember, we function like a symphony.

As you embark on a lifestyle change, remember what we talked about in chapter 3: small steps, even embarrassingly small steps. It's about building on successes, however small. If you fail to achieve your goal, it was too ambitious. Forget the setback and set a new goal that you can achieve, and remember—*no goal is too small.* Creating stress and anxiety over your goals will only add another threat and torpedo your efforts. Be patient. Allow yourself time. It's about a lifestyle change. Changing how you live your life. That's big and, by definition, takes time. Be kind, yet unwavering in your desire to adopt your new lifestyle. If you are patient and persistent, it will happen, and you will find that living a lifestyle that makes you stronger will become your new normal—easy and rewarding and empowering.

And remember, life has a sense of humor, and perhaps a sense of injustice, so plan on life throwing you a curveball. *It will come,* usually unannounced and without fanfare. One day you're on top of the world, all systems go, and the next minute, you're not, and life can change forever. How it changes; how much it changes; whether we're worse or better, weaker or stronger, still on track or sliding into decline—it all comes down to our *resilience.*

Resilience is the holy grail of successful aging. In physics, resilience is defined as a material's ability to resume its original shape or position after being bent, stretched, or dented. To age successfully, then, is to do all we can to avoid being "bent, stretched, or dented" and to bounce back when we are. Resilience, in human terms, is the ability to quickly recover from illness, change, or misfortune. The MacArthur Study first helped us realize the importance of lifestyle to aging successfully. Subsequent research has consistently and overwhelmingly validated this view. The right lifestyle gives us resilience. Resilience is about toughness. So use the Ten Tips to hone a lifestyle that will give you the tools, support, and understanding to take life's curveballs and hit them out of the park—or at least to not strike out when life calls you up to bat.

USE IT OR LOSE IT

Either you're growing or you're dying,
trying to get better or just trying to maintain.
If you only try to maintain, then you take away
any reason to do anything better.

—LOU HOLTZ

If you think you can do a thing, or you think you
can't do a thing, you're right.

—HENRY FORD

During the 1960s, when the country was bound together in the exciting quest to land a man on the moon, we watched with wonder as America's finest risked their lives to venture into the unknown, and in so doing they captured our admiration and became modern-day heroes. On several of the Apollo missions, however, we were shocked to see astronauts, recently plucked from their floating capsules, carried off the rescue helicopter on stretchers. We had to wonder, as indeed NASA did, what was it about space that, in just a matter of days, caused these highly screened and trained space athletes to become casualties?

We knew little of space and theorized all kinds of science-fiction explanations for what was happening. In fact, we know now that the

Soviet cosmonauts had experienced similar difficulties on returning to earth after long missions and frequently had to be carried from landing sites in reclining chairs. In time, NASA determined that lengthy exposure to zero gravity—to weightlessness—was the culprit.

You're in space, in weightlessness. Your world is now limited to just a few square feet of livable space. If you wish to move from one side of that space to the other, all you need do is push lightly on a solid object and you will propel yourself to where you wish to go. You float effortlessly. No challenge. No sweat. Even if you do move, your arms and legs have no weight. So your muscles take a rest. Your heart, also a muscle, takes a rest, since the column of blood it has to pump weighs less. So these highly trained muscles and your efficient physiology aren't used much. And even your bones they now have no weight to support so they begin to leach out calcium and get less strong. What did your grandmother tell you? Use it or lose it. Exactly. So you return to earth. You have less muscle mass, as much as 1 percent less for each week in space,[1] and you're weaker. Your heart now has to suddenly do much more work, like pumping a column of blood up to your brain in order to stay conscious when you stand. You've lost the strength and efficiency you had just a couple of weeks before.

OK, so what does all this have to do with you, an earthbound creature? You don't plan to be in weightlessness much in your lifetime, right? Well guess what—we can create our own brand of earthbound weightlessness.

Debilitating bed rest

My first realization of the toxicity of disuse came in my medical-training days. When a patient was afflicted with severe back pain, we routinely placed them on strict bed rest. I mean strict. No getting up to use the bathroom. No sitting up in a chair. When these patients finally stood straight again after seven days lying in bed, they frequently became lightheaded. Several nearly fainted. They complained of weakness, flabby muscles, and lack of balance. Many also felt that their mental function was affected, feeling their ability to remember or to come up with the right word was not what it had been just a week before. Upon investigating, we could see a significant drop in blood pressure when they stood. Their hearts couldn't do the job they had been doing before the bed rest. Although we didn't then measure muscle strength, it was clear their muscles were smaller and weaker. These people had experienced a decline. Maybe their back was better, but not much else. In fact, we know now that just a week of strict bed rest is the equivalent of aging two years or more![2] The normal rate of loss of muscle mass is about 0.5 to 1 percent per year after age forty.[3] Add to that what comes with inactivity, and Houston, we have a problem.

But unless your lover leaves you, you probably don't plan to stay in bed a week (and if you get a new lover, your time there doesn't qualify as strict bed rest). Well, in fact, couch potatoes, armchair athletes, movie or sports-events addicts, and probably the majority of our workers today, who gaze into a computer screen for most of the day—as much as 70 percent of us—may very well be categorized as "sedentary" by the President's Council on Fitness, Sports & Nutrition.[4] This is our earthbound version of weightlessness, and we are therefore in the "lose it" red zone.

Now, granted, when the astronauts began moving about under one G of gravity back on earth, and after our back-pain patients began spending more time standing, they regained some of what they lost. But what if for decades we coast, using only a small fraction of what we are capable of? What if our lifestyles are such that we minimize what we ask of our muscles, and brain, and social skills, and hand-eye coordination, and reasoning, and problem solving? Do we lose those also if we don't use them? As my friend Patsy from Minnesota says, "You betcha." What we don't use tends to go the way of a discarded bicycle, left out in the elements. It basically rusts to the point where it is no longer usable. We lose the ability to do what we could before.

A personal experience with rust

When I was in college, I was smitten with a blonde folk singer. I would follow her anywhere. And I did—right off a cliff on a toboggan. Many operations, and months using crutches, later, I was well again. Or so I thought. Turns out the lower leg they spent so much time trying get back together was not quite right. My knee and ankle were out of alignment. So, many years later, I began to experience pain and increasing limitation of motion. My image of myself as a military guy, an athlete, and overall godlike figure was smashed. I became depressed. I was working out less, going out less, making fewer presentations, reading less, and becoming, as my wife said, "one big pain in the butt." As I did less, whether physical, intellectual, or social, I was more and more, day by day, unable to do what I had been able to do the week before. I was circling the drain on a self-perpetuating slide to more and more limitation and impairment.

A major part of my environment is my wife, Paula. She's no shrinking violet and this has its benefits. She reflected my downward spiral to me and "encouraged" me to seek out someone who could correct my lower-leg problem. I did, at the nearby world-class Brigham and Women's Hospital in Boston. There, a top surgeon with experience with my problem thought he could help me. The surgery was successful; I began to get stronger with rehabilitation. With the physical strength came a restored optimism, more exercise, more social encounters, and a renewed interest in work and life in general. I was, in fact, doing a reverse, and very positive, upward spiral.

Rust is a crouching predator

As the human species evolved over millennia, life was about survival, requiring constant physical work, movement, and use of whatever faculties we had that could ensure the success of the tribe or village. Since this is, in fact, the experience we humans have lived for over 99 percent of the time we've been on earth, it is understandable that our physiology is wired to use these skills. Whether our heart, muscles or our brains, anything, we tend to get better at something the more we use it.

We don't usually choose to not use something. Over my many years of counseling people on how to stay healthy and perform at their best, I've never heard anyone declare, "I think I'll let this skill wither by not using it." Rather, it sneaks up on them like a predator. Take the bicycle we left leaning against the house months or years ago. We intended to use it, but just never got around to it. Maybe we got a new car and preferred the faster and less tiring way of getting around. Or we got a new job and had less time to ride. Or maybe we hurt our leg and couldn't ride anymore. Whatever the reason, the result is the same: the bike rusts and eventually is unusable. And so it is with the many faculties we take for granted over many decades. They can disappear without a big announcement and we are one day surprised that we are not what we used to be.

Even though we may ignore skills for years, we still expect them to be there when we need them. But they may not be there. Once we could crouch down without pain. Once we could walk five miles without any difficulty. Once we could memorize a phone number immediately. Once we were the life of the party. Once we thought deeply about the meaning of life. But somewhere along the way, life happened.

We took a job where we moved less. Our schedules got busy and we had less time or inclination to grow physically, intellectually, or even socially. A painful joint may have caused us to use that joint less. Difficulty with hearing, or having to urinate frequently, or trouble with memory may have prevented us from socializing, and before we realized it, we were avoiding social interaction. When learning began to take a little more time, or required complete quiet or concentration, we stopped taking classes or just avoided learning situations altogether.

Our inability to do what we could do in our twenties or thirties or forties might cause us to not want to "embarrass" ourselves by engaging in that activity at all. If we are in a sedentary or intellectually stagnant environment, our peers may cause us to "move toward the mean"—i.e., to be more like the average person in the group rather than to continue to challenge ourselves and grow. When Dr. Ellen Langer, professor of psychology at Harvard, placed older men in an environment similar to when they were twenty years younger, the group began to act younger than those in normal environments.[5] Studies of obese young adults show that weight loss is influenced by the group you associate with.[6] On the other hand, it's been shown that obesity can be "contagious"—that is, more common in groups where members are obese.[7]

So whether it's inattention, embarrassment, or more pressing needs, when we no longer regularly use our skills or faculties, whether physical, mental, or social, those skills decline, rust, and eventually—without warning, fanfare, or any notice at all—they are unusable.

The mixed effects of modern technology

We modern humans have done marvelous things. The rate of development of technology has been so rapid that many of us are astounded by what is possible while our coworkers or family members only a few years younger consider it commonplace. We are clearly challenging our brains, learning how to use the magical tools, all while traditional ways of working, learning, communicating, and living are being changed forever, along with the skills that were associated with them.

We can readily observe this process of loss of the skills that were once so necessary for everyday life but that have now been rendered unnecessary by technology. Take reading maps, a skill rapidly vanishing with the easy availability of the GPS. Or reading analog clocks, a skill we're losing as digital clocks become dominant. The loss of some skills or experiences is more troublesome, however, such as experiencing nature firsthand rather than through iPads or computers.

Richard Louv, author and child-advocacy expert, calls the lack of nature in the lives of today's wired-in children a "nature-deficit disorder." In *Last Child in the Woods*, he links some disturbing childhood trends, including obesity, attention disorders, and depression, to this lack of a nature experience.[8] Even more troublesome is our threatened basic ability to communicate with each other by voice, gesture, and touch—the way we learned to do eons ago, the way we inherited from our ancestors—in a world dominated by emails, texts, Facebook, and Twitter.

So as our society strives for efficiency, the quickness and ease of accomplishment of nearly every task, there is a subtle but powerful value system telling us what the signs of success are: less work at a task, more things done for us, less sweating to get a task done. This seems to be an unexamined, unchallenged value, something very few would dispute. But is it necessarily a good thing that we do things easier, quicker, or with less physical or mental effort? Should I, in fact, have someone else spread my mulch, as my neighbor Steve suggested in chapter 1?

At first look it would seem so. But while our technology develops at an accelerating rate, the evolution of our body and mind lags behind. We have, in fact, a situation where we may lose attributes, abilities, and skills we may no longer need to navigate the world but that are still necessary for our health or well-being.

For example, take something as simple as walking. Our bodies have evolved over millennia with walking as the basic mode of transportation and body movement. Our physiology and optimum functioning requires regular motion in muscles and joints, and such motion is even necessary for our brain to function optimally (see Tip Three for more on this). The design of our cities and the availability of automobiles, moving walkways, drive-throughs, elevators, escalators, televisions, computers, and so much more have made it not only less desirable to walk but also less necessary. We have become a sedentary society and we are paying a high health price.

Lester, the "cockeyed optimist"

Lester is ninety-eight, vital, articulate, a piano player, and still driving. He lives in a retirement community with Masterpiece Living and is convinced that his life is a model for successful aging. He tells me he's been very fortunate in his life: meeting Sybil, his wife of sixty-five years; being transferred from his military unit just before they went to Guadalcanal and were "chopped to pieces"; "falling into" a community-college teaching opportunity after he was retired from his career with Shell Oil Company; and now, living in his current community. It's not that he's been spared the slings and arrows of life: he is still raw from the loss of Sybil two years ago, visiting her every morning in "Sybil's Corner" of his apartment. Being her caretaker for many years as she declined with diabetes and Alzheimer's disease took its toll, too. He is estranged from his grandsons and only great-grandson, and his unbounded enthusiasm for life is not always appreciated by peers who choose to stop growing and learning. But despite this, Lester unabashedly declares, "My mission in life is to do things for people. I feel a desire and an obligation to help others . . . because I can." And he takes that mission seriously. Every morning he brings the newspaper to a friend in the assisted-living area of his community and spends some moments in conversation with her, and he has assisted her in dealing with medical matters. He formed a nonagenarians club to celebrate these elders and to keep them engaged in the community. Lester was desperately isolated after Sybil died and helped to form a Guardian Angel Society, neighbors helping neighbors. He organized a popular lecture series because "it's never too late to learn!" And of course, because the piano helped him win over Sybil's heart, he plays regularly at community social events, still warming hearts and stirring memories.

There is no "woe is me" with Lester. In fact, he repeatedly told me how fortunate he has been, and still is, given his abilities, his health, and the opportunity to live in a Masterpiece Living community. He is determined to use his abilities while he has them and knows that he's more likely to keep them longer by using them. His daughter calls him her "cockeyed optimistic" (and given that he spent World War II in the South Pacific, it fits). With such optimism and sense of community and purpose, Lester will undoubtedly have to begin serious consideration of forming a centenarian club.

Life has curveballs in store for us: bunches of them. Even when we don't realize we're at bat. Having a pulse is being at bat all the time. How we age is a function of how we handle these curveballs, how we avoid at least some of them, and how we expect them without stressing over them. One of the ways we can avoid some of those "slings and arrows" or rebound when they hit us is to be in the best shape possible, at our "fighting weight." When we experience a threat to our physical self, for instance, like I did when I had my leg injury, do we meet it head-on with a robust intellectual, social, and spiritual strength that can get us back on track, or does it permanently derail us and begin us down a path to further decline? If the threat to our aging comes in another dimension—the intellectual, social, or even spiritual—will resilience in these other dimensions help us to prevail no matter what we encounter in our magnificent journey through our lives?

Perhaps the analogy of riding horses is more useful to our understanding of this concept. When we fall, or get knocked out of the saddle, being strong in *all areas of our lives* can allow us to get back on and live with whatever adjustments we need to make. Living a healthy lifestyle, then, is about more than just being leaner, or better looking, or smarter, or able to do things others may not be able to. It's about *using and growing our skills, capabilities, and talents* so that we become as resilient as we can be in all areas of life, so that those threats we cannot avoid will not unseat us, will not take us out of the race. Rather, this resilience will allow us to be a survivor and to age successfully, to be as vital as we can possibly be, for as long as possible.

✍ *Masterpiece Living Pearls for Using It Before You Lose It*

1. Sit in a comfortable chair (just for a little while), put your feet up, and *think*. Picture yourself going through a typical day in five years: What does the day involve? How much walking? What brain and physical skills? How much strength? Resilience? Ability to read? What other people are involved?

2. Now picture yourself on a *special* day in five years: What brain, physical, and social skills will you be using?

    Example: Are you traveling? What does a travel day involve? How much walking? What tasks require strength? Balance? Ability to communicate? Ability to make your way in a foreign country or at higher altitude or in colder or warmer temperatures?

    Example: In your special-day scene, are you playing music or teaching or playing with your grandkids, or building something, or riding a bicycle? Again, what skills will you be using?

    Example: Are you doing something with a group? What group is it, and what are you doing together?

3. Now make a list of those skills used for both typical and special future days. Divide them up into physical, intellectual, and social skills.

    You have before you your immediate goals for your own successful aging. These are physical, intellectual, and social skills you must have to live the life you want to live. You may currently have the ability to walk, or the stamina to travel, or musical ability, or membership in a group; or you may not. In either case, *in order to be able to do these things in a month, a year, or five years from now, you will have to continue to use or develop these skills and abilities now.*

4. Make a personal lifestyle plan for each skill or ability. Remember, this is going to take some time. Be patient and realistic, and remember, *small steps*. Resist declaring a heroic goal and telling all your friends. Develop a plan—a pathway, really—where you will incorporate using or learning these desired abilities in your everyday life. It will be very advantageous to have a coach, someone who knows why you value cultivating these activities, skills, or abilities. Such a coach can guide you through rocky roads ahead, or merely remind you of why you made a lifestyle plan in the first place.

You will have to train like a warrior before a battle, a fighter for a fight, or an athlete before a championship game. The default situation, what will happen if you don't pay attention, is decline—losing. You're training for the fight of your life: the rest of your life. Your training is *using, refining, and even growing better skills.* Do that, and life will not take you to the metaphorical mat. Life's left hooks may knock you back on your heels sometimes. You may even get knocked down. But if you are the best that you can be physically, mentally, and socially, you will be more resilient and able to last the duration and be in charge of what this next phase of your life looks like. So put on the *Rocky* music, charge up the stairs, and raise your arms. You have what it takes to prevail, on your terms.

KEEP MOVING

*Movement is a medicine for creating change in a
person's physical, emotional, and mental states.*
—CAROL WELCH

Sitting is the new smoking.
—DR. JAMES LEVINE

What would you be willing to do to get the following outcomes: reduce the likelihood that you will be afflicted with heart disease, or stroke, or cancer, or diabetes, or dementia, or osteoporosis; reduce the likelihood that you will fall, and if you do fall, reduce the likelihood that you would break a bone; feel better; look better; and overall have more energy to enjoy life more? Sound good? Would you be willing to *move*? You're thinking there's got to be catch; there's something I'm not telling you, right? How and why can so many good things come from just moving?

No catch. It's true. It's simple, and only a few of us are doing it. A 2008 National Health Interview Survey study found that 36 percent of adults were considered inactive.[1] If we focus on older adults, that figure rises, along with the risk of—you guessed it—heart disease, stroke, cancer, diabetes, dementia, and osteoporosis. The same study found that 59 percent of adults never participated in vigorous physical activity lasting more than ten minutes in a given week.[2]

In a 2000 review in the *Journal of Applied Physiology*, Frank W. Booth, Scott E. Gordon, Christian J. Carlson, and Marc T. Hamilton pulled no punches and signaled that they take this very seriously. "Make no mistake," their review begins, "our society, and even the world's population in general, is truly at war against a common enemy. That enemy is modern chronic disease."[3] And in a later piece discussing the review, Dr. Booth and Manu V. Chakravarthy tell us that we're facing a "silent enemy": "sedentary lifestyle."[4] Their point is that man has a basic requirement to be physically active in order to be healthy; that he has inherited this from his ancestors; and that the rise of chronic disease has resulted in more sedentary lifestyle, which in turn results in more chronic disease. This is a threat to the lives and welfare of this country and, in fact, the globe.

Dr. James Levine of the Mayo Clinic-Arizona State University Obesity Solutions Initiative agrees. He tells us that "sitting is the new smoking." Yes, indeed the following is a list of the bad news:

SEDENTARY LIVING INCREASES THESE CONDITIONS

✓ Angina, heart attack, coronary artery disease

✓ Breast cancer

✓ Colon cancer

✓ Congestive heart failure

✓ Depression

✓ Gallstone disease

✓ High blood triglyceride

✓ High blood cholesterol

✓ Hypertension

✓ Less cognitive function

✓ Low blood HDL

✓ Lower quality of life

✓ Obesity (difficulty with weight control)

✓ Osteoporosis

✓ Pancreatic cancer

✓ Peripheral vascular disease

✓ Physical frailty

✓ Premature mortality

✓ Prostate cancer

✓ Sleep apnea

✓ Stiff joints

✓ Stroke

✓ Type 2 diabetes[5]

Booth estimates that physical inactivity accounts for approximately 15 percent of the entire healthcare costs of the United States.[6] His solution? The same as the recommendation of the Expert Panel of the Centers for Disease Control and of the American College of Sports Medicine: "Every US adult should accumulate 30 minutes or more of moderate-intensity physical activity on most, and preferably all, days of the week. . . . Adults who engage in moderate-intensity physical activity—i.e., enough to expend 200 calories per day—can expect many of the health benefits described [in this report]."[7]

So why are so many of us sedentary, and why is being sedentary so bad for us? Let's start with the last question. Sure, we all know that exercise is good for us. But let's not even use the "E" word. Moving is astoundingly good for us. Ken Cooper, the "father of aerobics" and founder of the Cooper Institute and the Cooper Clinic in Dallas, Texas, recently said in an interview that walking just two miles three or four times a week "would reduce deaths from heart attacks, strokes, diabetes, and cancer by 58 percent, and could potentially prolong life up to six years." Cooper, so long the advocate of running, is clear in his appreciation for the fine pastime most of us can do without instruction, special clothes, dedicated facilities, or even good weather. That pastime? Walking. Again, why is it that being sedentary is deadly?

Moving to survive

Let's go back to our ancestors again, back before elevators, escalators, cars, and even horses. This is when our human physiology was coming of age. Our ancestors had to move to survive. Not unlike most other mammals, humans had to expend much energy in order to acquire food and water. These early humans, with whom we share most of our physiology, were nomadic, and therefore moving was an essential part of their lives.

As descendants of these nomadic people, our physiology is based on abundant movement and a diet of vegetables, fruits, nuts, fish, and infrequent, small portions of meat (see Tip Five). To the extent we have that, we are more likely to be healthy. To the extent we don't, problems arise.

If you look at photos of crowds just over half a century ago, before *exercise* was a word, before the term *jogging* had meaning, before fitness centers, and before the hundreds of diet plans, you'll see that the people in these photos are lean. Almost every person—lean. Movement was an inherent part of daily life—walking, biking, work, play—and obesity was rare. Not exactly like our distant ancestors, but closer than we are today.

But today, we have virtually programmed physical movement out of daily life. We drive to work, drive through for our coffee, take an elevator or escalator to our office, sit at a computer or in meetings for the day, order out for lunch. Even laborers, although still moving more, are assisted with power tools instead of hand tools, crane baskets instead of ladders, and backhoes instead of shovels, and therefore move a little less. Most jobs involve sitting, lots of sitting.

Our children catch the school bus, which, as anyone who gets stuck behind one will tell you, stops every hundred feet to pick up a child who has been waiting in the family car parked at the bus stop with Mom. In school, physical education is deemphasized. After hours, we drive our kids where they need to be, and watch helpless as they spend countless hours sitting with computers, phones, and video players, or in front of the television.

How did all this happen? Those of us who lived through the fifties remember that "progress" and "success" usually meant easier (i.e., less physical) work. To the extent you were successful, you were able to obtain things that made it less necessary to walk, or open a garage door, or grow your own vegetables, or open a can. Leisure became inextricably attached to progress and success. Add to that the explosion of automobiles and then the age of technology, which changed workplaces and created huge industries where workers sat while at work.

Six decades later, movement, if it occurs at all, is scheduled. It's "working out." This concept of movement as an event rather than a lifestyle is, I believe, precisely why so few of us do it. Who has the time to work out? What more can I put into an already fully scheduled day? David Gobble, my good friend and colleague and the former director of the Fisher Institute for Wellness and Gerontology at Ball State University, shared with me a photo that he thought symbolized this removal of movement from our daily lives. Picture the front of a fitness center—with an escalator taking you up one flight of stairs!

This concept of movement as working out has resulted in a billion-dollar industry offering equipment, clothing, workout facilities, food, drinks, travel, and more, all geared to meeting our body's innate requirement for movement, and all distancing us, particularly those of us who are older, from the idea that movement is a natural state for us humans. And of course, what has further distanced us is the virtual explosion of fitness experts, programs, and approaches to fitness. This is an area lending itself to zealots, who usually offer a very prescriptive program with often unrealistic expectations, offering abundant opportunity for disillusionment.

Last, and probably most disruptive to a lifestyle of movement as way of life, is, ironically, the fact that movement, now tied to a fitness industry, is even more tightly tied to weight loss. Outside of training for athletic events or perhaps the military, weight loss and vanity are clearly the major reasons for attempting anything physical at all. If we lose the weight, we frequently lose the motivation to continue moving, and weight returns. If we don't lose the weight, we give up trying and the more frequent movement with it.

Now, before you cry foul, I am absolutely supportive of efforts to maintain a lean body, of the benefits of workouts, and of the culture of health and activity that is attached to our collective approach to movement. I believe the rehabilitative and fitness industries are filled with highly motivated professionals who work virtual miracles every day for injured, challenged, or otherwise impaired people. My criticism has to do with the fact that this technology-based, highly prescriptive approach leads one to believe that movement *must* be managed by science, *must* involve specific machines or approaches, and *must* result in weight loss to be of value.

These characteristics have value, but they are obstacles when viewed as absolute necessities for bringing physical activity into our lives. Looking at the endless supply of programs, exercise machines, clothing, diets, and consultants easily pushes most people past the threshold for fear. And fear will never work as a long-term motivator.

So, ironically—and tragically—as movement became detached from our lifestyles, there arose the need for the fitness industry, which, when seen as the only way to be physically active, further distances movement from our basic lifestyles (a self-perpetuating situation). Movement—walking, for instance—can be free and highly effective for keeping us healthy. Cost, complexity, fear, or lack of familiarity with physiology should not be deterrents to beginning a lifestyle of movement.

What's really killing us?

As we noted previously, the Centers for Disease Control has identified heart disease, cancer, lung disease, strokes, and Alzheimer's disease as the major chronic-disease killers of Americans.

- But if you ask them what's *really* killing us (wink, wink) they will tell you another story. They will tell you that, overwhelmingly, it is conditions that are related to lifestyle that kill us:

- Smoking: 400,000

- Diet and activity patterns (sedentary lifestyle, calorie-rich foods): 300,000

- *Alcohol: 100,000* [8]

We can see, then, that modifiable behavior—lifestyle—is indeed a major factor in how and why we die, and, as noted by the MacArthur Study, how well we age. Physical inactivity, with its ties to obesity, heart disease, cancer, stress, mood, and our immune system, plays a leading role in this tragedy.

If I were king

It's rare indeed that there is one solution to many problems. But it does happen. The problems of heart disease, stroke, many cancers, obesity, diabetes, osteoporosis, depression, and dementia are multifactorial in their causes but *all* are positively affected by physical activity. Unfortunately, as we mentioned above, *physical activity—movement—has been systematically removed from the daily life of most of us.* It has been replaced by excellent alternatives (fitness centers, jogging, classes, home exercise machines), but all of these are add-ons to our already full lives. If I were king, or at least had the ability to change one thing to positively affect the health, aging, and overall quality of life for all, I would bring walking (or biking) back into the fabric of our lives; redevelop cities, workplaces, and neighborhoods to allow all to walk or bicycle as they go about their daily lives, doing errands, going to meetings, going to movies or out to eat.

As Dan Buettner tells us in his Power 9® observations from the Blue Zones, we should move naturally like Blue Zone inhabitants who live in environments that constantly nudge them into moving without thinking about it. They grow gardens and don't have mechanical conveniences for house and yard work.[9]

In fact, if we are to be truly healthy, movement should occur throughout the day rather than be scheduled. There are now concerns that even those who may have regular workouts, but then spend the rest of the day sitting, are still at risk.

"Avoiding sedentary time and getting regular exercise are both important for improving your health and survival," said Dr. David Alter, Senior Scientist, Toronto Rehab, University Health Network (UHN), and Institute for Clinical Evaluative Sciences. "It is not good enough to exercise for 30 minutes a day and be sedentary for 23 and half hours."[10]

Movement is, for us as a species, closer to our real selves, our authentic selves. Awareness of the potential for this lifestyle is growing, and more and more planned cities and neighborhoods are designing better alternatives to our too-dangerous-to-walk cities and neighborhoods. Many initiatives, like the Robert Wood Johnson Foundation's Active Living by Design (www.activelivingbydesign.com), are working with communities to bring about this type of substantial change.

The rest of us cannot afford to wait. We all have a responsibility for our own health. Even the smallest of changes can result in marked reduction in risk and higher quality of life.

Movement as a lifestyle

OK. You agree that movement is important. Before you rush to the store and to get your Under Armour exercise clothing, let's be reasonable about this. If this is going to work, it must be a lifestyle change. If it is something that is going to be resilient and outlast the slings and arrows of our crazy frenetic lives (and it must!), then this is not something to take lightly. This is as great a *lifestyle* change as deciding to go back to school, or moving to a new city, or getting divorced (not really that last one, but I wanted to impress on you that it's big). Remember the concept of kaizen. Then decide what *small* change you're going to make. Teresa, my no-nonsense colleague, sent me a reminder: "If you change nothing, nothing will change." Remember, small. If you decide to walk five minutes, or ten, or fifteen, do it with a friend, two legs or four; both will become embedded in your prefrontal cortex and make you want to do the right thing. And perhaps that is the best way to begin. Walking. No equipment, no special facilities, no need for trumpets and fanfare to begin.

Now let me predict what will happen. You will begin. You will feel good about yourself although you will have a tendency to say "I'm only . . ." *Don't do that!* No apologies. You're beginning. You're better off than perhaps as much as a third of our population. The only failure here is the failure to try. You'll begin to think either (1) *This is silly, why don't I start training for a marathon (or something bigger than what I'm doing)?* or (2) *This is silly, it can't be helping.*

Can't be helping? Really? After all I've told you, and in spite of the fact that you *do* feel better? So keep it up. Don't listen to the critic in your mind. Listen instead to your body. Become aware, as you walk and move, of how that feels. Pay attention to how you're sleeping, thinking, and feeling. Pay attention to your energy level. Your level of stress and anxiety. All will improve. This will happen. There is a marvelous line from the movie *The Best Exotic Marigold Hotel*: "Everything will be all right in the end. If it's not all right, it's not yet the end." The more you become aware of your body, and of your inner self, the more you will feel the truly magnificent changes happening to you.

You will persist. You will increase what you are doing. The main challenge will be to resist the impulse to "go Olympic" and try to take on too much. Remember, this is a about lifestyle alteration, not training. Training has an inherent element of time limitation. I'll train until the event. Then I'm not training anymore. Your change is timeless. Your new self. Your new lifestyle.

Where does it all lead?

This all leads to a daily lifestyle that includes sleeping, eating, *movement*, and all the other particulars of your life. Movement every day. Movement that you enjoy. Maybe eventually you'll add things like biking, or swimming, or gardening for that thirty minutes. Maybe you'll even join a fitness center! Who knows? But it will be out of a joy of movement, not out of guilt or desire to conquer the world, or because you want bragging rights with your friends at the diner downtown. If for some reason you truly cannot walk or work up to being able to walk, then assess what you can do: chair exercises, sitting yoga, or many other creative things that are possible in your home.

If you are to enjoy the platinum plan of movement, you will add flexibility and balance movements, like yoga, or tai chi, or just plain stretching. Or not. You will add strength movements, like hand weights, or bands, or actual strength machines. Or not. Maybe you will or maybe you won't, but it's *not a prerequisite to becoming better through movement in your life*. Just move. Don't put it on your to-do list. Make it the paper, your basic life, that the to-dos are added to. Nonnegotiable. The stuff of your life.

And you will reap the horn of plenty from your new lifestyle: lowered blood pressure and lipids; improved cardiovascular efficiency and lung function; less joint pain; improved balance and resilience; lowered risk for all the major threats to our successful aging experience, including heart attacks, strokes, cancer, dementia, and diabetes; better mood; sharper thinking; better sleep; less body fat; better looks . . . well, OK, maybe not, but I guarantee you will be told by those around you that you look good. Your body will be just overjoyed with what you are doing and will release brain substances, like dopamine, endorphins, serotonin, all of which will make you feel on top of the world. No magic, just the entire body-mind-spirit responding to what it needs and craves and finding its true nature in your new lifestyle of movement.

Dorothy dared

Dorothy was in her seventies and had led a full life. She had retired after working in a medical office for decades, and enjoyed living in her home and adapting to her new life as a retired person. But now, after a decade of retirement, she knew she was in trouble. She had severe knee pain, had gained weight, and now had diabetes. She also knew that she had become more isolated over her decade of retirement. So she dared.

She dared to move from her home of so many years into a retirement community. She did it to become more engaged with other people. She chose one that had Masterpiece Living and that offered her both the opportunity to evaluate her current lifestyle and the support to make the changes she chose to make. When she saw her Lifestyle Inventory feedback report, she was not surprised. She had little social engagement, was stagnant intellectually, and was doing little to nourish her inner self. But she knew immediately what she needed to attend to first. *She had to address her physical self first.*

She began modestly with water aerobics at 5:30 a.m. and met some marvelously animated people who were unafraid to put a bathing suit on again. She began walking regularly and soon found others who enjoyed walking and talking. She joined groups with the community and filled her day with social activity and more and more movement. She was much happier—and along the way, during that first year in her new life, some other things happened. She lost seventy pounds and returned to her high school weight. Her doctor told her she no longer had diabetes. And her knee no longer hurt! She was active, engaged, and fulfilled. She felt empowered, with a new lease on life, and she dared more. She dared to take up the flute again after forty years. She dared to start a small musical group that actually played in public! Dorothy dared to move, and it made all the difference.

❧ Masterpiece Living Pearls for Keeping Moving

Get out a small book and pen. Now make sure you have it with you at all times over the next three days. You're going to keep track of how you spend your day, with a focus on how much you move, or don't. Next, get a pedometer. You can get one in Target or Walmart or a sporting-goods store. You're going to have this with you at all times, hooked on your belt at the hip, because it's going to tell you how many steps you take in a day or, if you want to know, how far you walk during an average day (multiply the number of steps you take by the length of your step). The directions that come with the pedometer will guide you. *Don't cheat!* You're getting a real baseline of your current movement, which will serve as a baseline from which you can grow. It's crazy to do more than you usually do. You can start that in a few days after you have a realistic assessment of just how much movement is currently in your life.

1. Now, take a look at your notes and number of steps per day. It's time to set your first goals. After three days of counting steps, figure out your average number of steps per day (take the total for that period and divide by three). Now how much do you want to increase that for the next week? *That's too much!* No matter what you said, I bet it is

too much for a first goal. Remember. *Small increases.* Add 1 percent (take the total and divide by 100), or 2 percent or 3 percent, to your average for the last three days and shoot for that for each day over the next week. See how that feels. Be proud when you do it. Check your total during the day to see if you need to step it up a bit to meet your goal. Reevaluate your goals each week and raise or lower them based on a realistic evaluation of how it's working for you.

2. At the same time, look at your notes of how you spend your time. How much is spent sitting, riding, or in general not moving? Perhaps an easy beginning is to stand while you're watching TV or work-ing with the computer, and walk in place. Get some steps on your pedometer. Even if just for a few minutes. No sweat, only move-ment. Where else in your day might you begin to think of move-ment as an essential part of your routine: like eating, sleeping, or dressing. What part of your routine can you now rethink in order to ensure that there is nonnegotiable time for purposeful movement? Start with only a few minutes and build on it as it feels right. Shoot to work up to thirty minutes and then see where that leads you. It will be easier than you think. Try walking the dog, or walking while you talk on the phone. Park farther from the store. Take at least one flight of stairs before you use the elevator. Try walking as you attempt to solve a problem.

3. If you have significant limitations to your ability to move, do what you can and make a commitment to add to it with small increments. You'll be surprised what you can do. If at any time you feel unwell or have pain, stop what you're doing until you feel better. If the feelings return even when you do less, then see your doctor for some guid-ance. Even those with significant disease can improve their physical self. It just may take longer or involve some accommodations.

4. Do those things for a month or two and see what happens. Take note of how much you increase your movement. How much better your mood, joints, and overall quality of life are. Don't even bother to weigh yourself. Weight might come off or it might not *but you are getting healthier!* Remember, this isn't about numbers or pant size or bragging rights. This is about changing your lifestyle to include more movement that will ensure you will age more successfully. You will stay independent longer. You will enjoy life more.

5. As you begin to notice remarkable improvements, pay attention to them and celebrate them. Just regroup if you don't meet a goal. Decide whether that goal was too ambitious and just reboot, so to speak. Focus on your successes, your improvements. This is the beginning of a magnificent adventure—really—to a life you've always wanted and now are beginning to realize you can achieve. All it takes is patience with yourself. Resistance to that voice in your head that says you should be doing more. More will come and you will know when it's time. More movement. Different types of movement—flexibility, balance, strength. Maybe doing some things you never thought possible . . . or maybe not. As long as you are moving more, you are growing, becoming healthier, and connecting with your core human needs and what it takes to be authentically healthy. You will also be making a substantial investment in your future, which will pay huge dividends. There's no going back. This is your new life, and it's awesome!

CHALLENGE YOUR BRAIN

I have no special talents.
I am only passionately curious.
—ALBERT EINSTEIN

How did the scarecrow know he didn't have a brain?
—LANCE W. BLEDSOE

*I*n the 1967 Mike Nichols film, *The Graduate*, Dustin Hoffman plays Ben Braddock, a recent college graduate, who gets one word of advice from a family friend: "Plastics."

Why? Because at the time, it was an exploding field with great potential. Over five decades later, if we look for a similar word representing an exploding field with great potential, it's *neuroplasticity*.

Neuroplasticity "refers to the lifelong capacity of the brain to change and rewire itself in response to the stimulation of learning and experience."[1] Or said another way, "the brain's ability to reorganize itself by forming new neural connections throughout life. Neuroplasticity allows the neurons in the brain to compensate for injury and disease and to adjust their activities in response to new situations or to changes in their environment."[2]

If you're not up out of your chair yelling "What!" then read this definition again. "Change and rewire itself . . . in response to . . . learning . . . or to changes in their environment . . . compensate for injury . . . throughout life!" This is heady stuff indeed and from my point of view can make the difference between a life of worry that I'm going to end up with everyone around me rolling their eyes because I've "lost it" and one where I can mix it up intellectually with the best of them even when I'm in my tenth decade of life. This is big.

And so is the whole field of brain health. The field of brain fitness is exploding, much like my own brain as I try to distill the critical components of what this all means. Basically, the idea that the adult brain is a relatively stagnant and fragile organ is no longer accepted. The brain changes throughout life, and we are, in fact, the architects. And so, once again, we have a lot to do with not only how our body ages but also how our brain ages.

Becoming your own Department of Transportation

Think of the brain as a collection of millions of miles of roads. In fact, that's what the brain is: roughly 100,000 miles of neural pathways. And every time we wish to move, learn something new, recall a fact, recognize someone, or do any of the magnificent things our brain is capable of, messages travel along these pathways at hyper-speeds of up to nearly three hundred miles per hour and enable us to do the task we wish.

OK. Say you learn something new. Whatever, the list of presidents, or how to play "Mr. Tambourine Man" on the guitar. Now think of that list or skill as a destination—say, Boston—where you want to go. Once you've learned it, you have built a neural pathway to Boston. Keep doing it and you build a neural freeway to Boston so you can get there faster (do it better). Stop doing it and the road you built gets smaller, and eventually some bridges will wash out, or it gets potholes and you can't get there as fast, or at all (can't do it as well, or at all). Say you want to learn something new. You want to go to New York instead. Again, you'll build a path, then a freeway, and as long as you *use it*—you guessed it—*you won't lose it*. Don't use the road and you will lose it.

What happens if something wipes out the road you built, say a head injury or a stroke? You will not be able to travel that road and do what you did before, whether it's speaking, or walking, or remembering your first dog's name. But what if you want to do those things? What if you work at it? You got it. In many cases, somehow the brain will find a route around the damaged area to your destination. That's neuroplasticity, the brain rewiring in response to the environment and a behavior.

When Dr. Jill Bolte Taylor was thirty-seven and a neuroanatomist at Harvard, she had a stroke that left her unable to speak, walk, or do much of anything she had done before as an intellectual. She describes her remarkable journey in her book *My Stroke of Insight*.[3] Her story is compelling on many levels, but what is particularly astonishing for all of us is that after eight years, she was fully recovered. After a long road of rehabilitation and dogged determination, she walks, writes, and speaks publicly about her experiences. Of course, her catastrophic cerebral hemorrhage wiped out part of her brain, destroying many of her pathways. But, determined to regain what she lost, she has clearly built new roads, either by finding other routes to her goal and building those up, or perhaps, even by making new ones. By a process called axonal extension, neurons are able to grow connections to other brain cells to create a pathway. Other neuron appendages, called dendrites, which bring signals into the neuron, are also able to grow and create or enlarge new pathways.

And Jill Bolte Taylor's story, despite its dramatic outcome, is not an outlier. Returning soldiers from Iraq and Afghanistan with devastating brain injury have shown a remarkable ability to recover. The ABC television journalist Bob Woodruff, injured by a roadside bomb in Iraq, is a well-known example of these new possibilities.

It's all good news

When I was in medical school, the prevailing belief was that once we were physically at maturity, we no longer made new brain tissue. After our brains were fully formed, aging and all the situations associated with aging (i.e., head trauma, hypoxia, heart attacks) gradually depleted the neurons in our brain, causing the brain to atrophy until we succumbed to senile dementia. That's what we all believed just a few decades ago. And, fortunately, we were wrong.

What we have now that we didn't have then is the ability to scan functioning brains, to look at brains as they are working! This has given us remarkable ability to better understand brain function, response to challenge, and reaction to specific tasking, as well as anatomical information that we can now correlate with function. And what we've discovered is remarkable indeed, a very optimistic picture of what's possible and of our role in making those possibilities a reality.

First of all, "use it or lose it" applies to the brain function as well as to the body. When we use the skills and knowledge we have, the pathways, the many connections within the brain, like the roads we spoke of earlier, remain functional and in the best shape they can be. Don't use them, and they become more difficult to use if not completely unusable. In fact, by a process called synaptic pruning, the connections making up the unused pathway atrophy—basically go away. Areas of the brain can atrophy when the functions they are responsible for are no longer or rarely used. In fact, atrophy of the brain is a common observation with aging, but what used to be an accepted part of getting older is now in question. Is the atrophy of aging merely the result of lack of use? The answer seems to be, for the most part, a resounding *yes*! So, if we continue doing those crossword puzzles, playing that guitar, speaking a second language, making that furniture, or cooking our favorite pasta, we continue to do it well. This equates to basic maintenance of our brain function and essentially involves staying engaged with things we have always done.

But there's more good news. It's clear that, under certain conditions, not only is the brain able to make new connections by means of extending connections with the parts of the cells called axons and dendrites, but the brain is also able to make *new cells*! This is indeed much more optimistic information than we learned in medical school. Neurogenesis, the ability to make new neurons, is well documented in the mammalian brain and can persist well into old age. The solid evidence for new cell generation is currently limited to areas of the brain important for making new memory and converting that short-term memory to long-term memory, as well as the areas important for spatial navigation, the ability to get from one place to another. Within the memory area, the hippocampus, however, it appears that although new cells appear, not all survive, and that stress and depression decrease neurogenesis. The hippocampus, in fact, is one of the first areas affected by Alzheimer's, bringing into question the role of depression and stress in the development of the disease. There is growing evidence for neurogenesis occurring in other areas of the brain, such as the cerebellum, responsible for movement coordination. Recent research has linked meditation to more gray matter and to less age-related atrophy of the brain.[4]

Brain scans can tell us what is happening as the brain works. People learning new skills, such as a language, show activity and, over time, growth in areas of the brain where these skills reside. Brains get larger in areas housing the new skill. It appears that we are indeed the architects of our own brain. Challenge it, and it will respond.

What is the significance of brain growth? First, it tells us that the brain is alterable, and not some static organ that is gradually declining. Second, this ability to grow—this neuroplasticity and neurogenesis—allows us to learn new things no matter what our age. Third, although there is not yet clear evidence that we can prevent or cure Alzheimer's, there is a growing body of evidence that suggests we can influence our risk of developing symptoms of this dreaded disease. How? You guessed it. Lifestyle.

The nuns would have none of it

A long-term study in Minnesota involved tracking the lifestyles and mental decline in a group of nuns.[5] When they died, autopsies showed some with Alzheimer's brains; there were tangles of neurons, and the plaques of beta amyloid material surrounded many neurons. Yet, prior to their death, these nuns had experienced no symptoms of Alzheimer's. No significant memory loss, no agitation or withdrawal. Basically, the brain pathology was a surprise to all and warranted a theory of explanation. The investigators concluded that a lifestyle of regular physical and mental activity protected the individual from the onset of symptoms even when the disease was present anatomically. These intriguing conclusions have been validated by subsequent research and are the basis for new approaches to brain health. In fact, two recent studies reported that dementia rates in Britain and Denmark have dramatically declined over the last two decades—observations attributed by the researchers to better healthcare and changing social factors such as education.[6]

In fact, neuroplasticity, neurogenesis, and the potential for preventing dementia make up an extremely active field of research, media stories, and a wave of new products claiming brain health as an outcome. So, with the overpowering amount of claims and products out there, what is fact and what, if anything, can we do to make it more likely we will not fall victim to dementia?

Fact and fiction: The gray of gray matter

What we do know is that the brain is a dynamic organ and can remain that way even as we age. We know that we can continue to learn as long as we have a pulse. Clear also, thanks to brain imaging, is that the brain has the ability to respond to environment, behavior, and even disease and devastating injury. This knowledge of the brain's ability to rewire itself and make new cells—in other words, of neuroplasticity and neurogenesis—has rewritten the books on what is possible as we age. Lowering the likelihood of falling victim to declining cognitive function, however, requires that we once again act as warriors against the threats to our mental function: cardiovascular disease, stress, cognitive laziness, and injury. Fortunately, these threats can all be dramatically reduced by how we choose to live our lives, by our lifestyle, by the choices we make every day. You do have a say in how well your brain will age. So, what is that lifestyle?

Once again, it's clear that we must pay attention to all aspects of our life in order for our brain to function at its best and remain healthy longer. The Ten Tips in this section, in fact, all relate to our brain as well as to the rest of our body. We are one organism, and although science and medicine have fractionated us into neurologic, cardiovascular, gastrointestinal, and a multiplicity of systems, in order to deal with the vast amount of information known about each, we move through life, get sick or stay healthy, and eventually die as one organism. All aspects of us relate and interact with each other. One affects the other, whether positively or negatively, and so we ignore aspects of our whole self—our core, authentic, species-driven self—only at great peril. So, knowing this, we are not surprised to hear what lifestyle qualities are associated with a better cognitive aging experience. Dr. Rob Winningham, a colleague of mine from Western Oregon University, authored a book called *Train Your Brain: How to Maximize Memory Ability in Older Adults.* This book is one of the more comprehensive and well-researched books on the topic, and strongly advocates lifestyle as an effective approach to continued brain fitness.[7]

Dr. Winningham is not alone in his focus on lifestyle. Brain-fitness experts agree on which lifestyle characteristics deliver the goods when it comes to cognitive function:

1. **Physical activity.** Neuroplasticity and neurogenesis cannot occur without the oxygen and glucose in blood. Our neurons cannot function without nutrients. Brain damage due to loss of blood supply can be devastating. Physical activity is associated with a surge of substances that stimulate brain growth. Brain-derived neurotrophic factor (BDNF) is like Miracle-Gro for the brain, as is nerve growth factor (NGF). Experiments in mammals have shown that these substances can reverse age-related memory impairments.[8]

2. **Mental stimulation.** The brain is no exception to the "use it or lose it" mantra. Neuroplasticity and effective neurogenesis will not occur unless the brain is stimulated by environment or behavior. That's us. That's us using our brain, and challenging it to keep the connections it has and to grow more. Learning new things and keeping our level of brain activity up is a virtual fountain of youth. The creative arts are particularly powerful sources of stimulation as well as source of healthy mindfulness.

3. **Stress control.** The chronic stress that is accepted as part of living in our modern world is, among other adverse effects, destructive to our cognitive function and raises our risk of dementia. The answer is not multitasking or drinking more coffee or working harder. It is finding those moments of awareness without thought, peace without chattering mind. It is connecting with others, whether human or animal, and experiencing the depth and joy of being; and it is being physical and getting the sleep you need to mend and grow.

4. **Regularly unplugging.** Our technology has provided us with fantastic capabilities. One of them is multiple ways of communicating. However, always being plugged in is not being socially connected— it is being technologically constrained. We can easily become prisoners of our phones, texts, or emails. This creates a chronic stressful situation with all the negative effects on our brains (and whole bodies—see Tips Five and Seven). These new technologies make us think we can multitask. My esteemed colleague Dr. Sandra Chapman, founder and chief director of the Center for BrainHealth at the University of Texas at Dallas and author of *Make Your Brain Smarter*, advises us about the "power of one"—her point being that our brains are not wired to do two things at once. Instead of multitasking, she recommends we "sequential task."[9] Dr. Adam Gazzaley of the University of California, San Francisco, is a loud voice for the potential negative effects of multitasking on our memory, learning, relationships, and jobs. Interacting with our new, high-tech environment is a challenge, he tells us in *The Distracted Mind*, a PBS special.[10]

5. **Balanced nutrition.** High-fat diets, obesity, and foods that cause wide swings in blood glucose throw water on the fire of our mental function. As with so many of the body's function and risks, inade-

quate or imbalanced nutrition "starves" our cells of nutrients, the fuel we need to work, to work well, to stay healthy, and to grow. We are a miracle of eons of evolution and of the refinement of our mammalian processes. This miracle has needs that our mass production of food, and the easy availability of poor-quality foods, are more and more failing to meet. A study at the Johns Hopkins Bloomberg School of Public Health, in fact, suggests that the risk of dementia is 47 percent greater, and of Alzheimer's disease 80 percent greater, for people with obesity.[11]

And so it's once again clear. The road to excellent brain health is pretty much the road to overall health, and that road is a lifestyle that pays attention to our physical, spiritual, and social health as well as the intellectual. It's not a difficult concept; it's not as difficult as you might think. There are undoubtedly people in your life who are doing it. Take Nola, for example.

Nola knows

Nola is a celebrity of sorts in the world of successful aging. She will tell you she was born in 1911, but she says, "I don't keep track of my age." Widespread recognition came when she earned her college degree at age ninety-five. That was, in fact, a world record, but she went even further, earning her master's degree at age ninety-eight.

Nola raised four sons with her husband, Vernon, on a family farm. When her husband died in 1972, she began taking college courses. When she was within thirty credits of completing her degree, she moved a hundred miles to a university apartment to finish alongside Alexandra, one of her thirteen grandchildren. Governor Kathleen Sebelius of Kansas presented the degree to her, an event that was followed by appearances on *The Early Show*, MSNBC, CBS News, and *The Tonight Show with Jay Leno*.

After her undergraduate diploma ceremony, Nola fulfilled a dream of being a storyteller on a cruise ship when she took a job as a guest lecturer for a nine-day Caribbean cruise. And of course, Alexandra went also. Before pursuing her master's, she of course took time to help with the family wheat harvest.

So, it's no wonder Nola is a rock star of successful aging! It's all there: the physical, intellectual, social, purpose, growing, scaring yourself, intergenerational contact—all with a smile that lights up a room. I'm reminded of pop culture rallying cries of "No fear" and "No limits." Yes, Nola is a successful ager and I can only imagine what her brain looks like.

❧ *Masterpiece Living Pearls for Challenging Your Brain*

1. Take a walk. If you do one thing for your brain, walk—or ride a bike, or swim. Do anything that gets you moving again. Whatever it is, enjoy it, and to keep doing it, walk or bike or swim with a friend. The point is, get blood flowing into the nooks and crannies of that magnificent control center called your brain. That brain you are designing and remodeling every day. Remember, start small. Very small. Miniscule. Just keep building on your successes, and if you fail just take a step back and begin succeeding again. Take a month or more to accumulate a mile of walking if necessary. There is no standard. Only you beginning and then continuing to move. There are huge gains with a small investment.

2. When you get back from your walk, *learn something new*. Be a beginner. What would you attempt if you knew you couldn't fail? What have you always wanted to learn or attempt? Forget about becoming an expert. Forget about how long it will take to learn. Strive to be a beginner. Be fearless in learning new things, doing things a little differently, scaring yourself a little every day. Ritual is a comforting and nurturing thing, but ritual is doing things mindfully, with awareness. If we do the same things without awareness, like a robot, it is not ritual, it's habit, and our brains are the equivalent of a bystander. Sure, continue doing those crossword puzzles, reading the paper, balancing your checkbook, but realize that it takes more to protect your brain from the ravages of time, stress, and lack of challenge. Engage your brain with new information, skills, pastimes. Learn how to order a meal in a different language; eat with the opposite hand; learn to make noise with a musical instrument or learn to play a new song on the instrument you do play; go to the grocery store a different way or go to a new grocery store. Forget about failing. *Not* trying new things is failure.

3. Realize that stress basically rots your brain. You, and only you, can shut the door on your particular brand of the Big Uneasy—stress. Joseph Campbell told us to find our bliss. That's it. Find what gives us joy, the feeling that comes from within where there's awareness

of this moment without thought. Painting, woodworking, nature walks, reading, music, children, knitting, meditation—seek out those things that quiet your chattering, stress-mongering mind. Find this quiet place within you and make sure you go there regularly to break the spell of your stress. You must be in charge.

And remember the role of moving, sleeping, social connection, and play in keeping the beast of stress at bay. Your brain will flourish. You will flourish. Those around you will feel your peace. You will live rather than endure.

4. Don't seek relief in the wrong places. You do want to quiet your chattering mind, but you do not want to disengage your brain. Even in restful sleep, we dream. Our brains are processing and reprogramming and recharging. When we watch television, it is as if our brains are on autopilot, as if we're drifting off to sleep or staring at a blank wall. Yes, we do need sleep and regular freedom from chattering mind, but seeking it in television, or drugs, or alcohol, or overeating is a dead end for our brains, and for some, a dead end for our lives.

5. All you need is love . . . and the right food. Our brains are only as good as the fuel we provide them. High-fat diets not only put us at high risk for heart disease, stroke, obesity, diabetes, and cancer, they also promote the development of Alzheimer's disease. Brains (and everything attached to our brains) function better on a diet of vegetables, fruits, fish, and whole grains (see Tip Five). Green, leafy vegetables are particularly a winner. The more a food has been altered for consumption (i.e., processed), the less valuable (and possibly more harmful) it is. Go fresh. Go local. If your great-grandmother never ate it, more than likely you shouldn't either.

6. Let your brain play. As mentioned before, Dr. Sandra Chapman tells us about the "power of none"[12]—basically, when you stop the chatter, your brain likes to experiment and creativity flourishes. To get an "aha moment," Chapman says, quiet your mind. Focus on a task that makes time "fly by" and makes you feel less stressed.

    Brain fitness is a field exploding, and a wide variety of "brain games" are flooding the market. Which games or approaches you use is a matter of personal taste. Look for those that have you learn something new and continue to challenge you with new tasks or facts. Just getting expert at one game has limited value. In the end, we want to treat our brains like a work of art, and we are the artist.

STAY CONNECTED

It's better to eat fries with friends, than broccoli alone.
—JOHN SPOONER

The Masai people of East Africa—whose "Life is change" maxim I cited earlier—have another saying: "We are not human unless we are with other humans." As we noted earlier, for most of the time we have walked the earth, we have walked with others. We did it for survival, and somewhere along the way, this basic need to be with others seems to have been encoded in our very DNA. We thrive with others. We seek out others. Of course, this need is consistent with the principle of nature that those characteristics associated with higher rates of survival are perpetuated. Our ancestors were extremely socially connected. It was an absolute necessity, and those who did not band with others did not survive.

We all can easily observe that, for the most part, we are happier with others. Yes, our fellow humans can sometimes make us want to tear our hair out. We can annoy each other, hurt each other, be less than noble to each other, but there remains a magnetic attraction that is deeper than personal preference. When faced with a choice between being alone or with others, most of us, most of the time, choose people. This is, again, at the core of our human needs, of our authentic self.

Robert Wright, journalist and author who writes about evolutionary psychology, uses game theory to cut to the chase of what drives human decision making. Game theory is a tool developed in the early twentieth century to study decision making. If, Dr. Wright tells us, game theorists were to apply their tools to human evolution, and therefore to basic human choices, there would be only three simple rules in this ultimate game.

First, the object of the game should be to maximize genetic proliferation. Second, the context of the game should mirror reality in the ancestral environment, an environment roughly like a hunter-gatherer society. Third, once the optimal strategy is found, the experiment isn't over. The final step—the payoff—is to figure out what feelings would lead human beings to pursue that strategy. Those feelings, in theory, should be part of human nature, should have evolved through generations and generations of the evolutionary game.[1]

As man was struggling to survive, with small numbers and a harsh environment, traits that led to the continuation of the species were desirable. Actually, they were more than desirable, according to Darwin—they were the traits that determined who would produce viable offspring and therefore would survive as a species. Anything that resulted in more chance for survival was passed on to offspring. Traits that hindered survival were lost with those who failed to survive. Many of those traits that did survive drive us to interact with others of our species.

Winning traits

Sexual attraction would, of course, be an obvious "feeling" and therefore a major component of human nature in this game. Sexual attraction, or at least opposite-gender attraction, is a major component of why we seem fascinated with others of our species. This powerful universal drive is also necessary for the propagation of our genes and therefore our survival as a species. Without this innate and, at times, all-consuming instinctual inclination to seek out the opposite sex, none of us would be here today. Probably next to the ability to seek out and find food, the instinct to procreate is preeminent. Surely, as mentioned earlier, we have come a long way, with a global population of over seven billion, but our instinctual traits change much more slowly, and so we are left with instincts that originated with our hunter-gatherer ancestors. As a species we remain drawn to the opposite gender, particularly during the years when procreation is possible, but to some extent for our entire lives.

Another successful trait for survival was the ability and inclination to be part of a group. If you were a loner, or for whatever reason were not able to assimilate into a group, your likelihood of survival (and of having offspring) was dramatically reduced.

Throughout our lives, we remain observers, joiners, and seekers of our own two-legged version of mammal. We love to watch each other in airports and on the street. We feel a deep satisfaction when we are part of a group, and deep discomfort when we are excluded. We are drawn to restaurants, sporting events, and other opportunities to be part of a group, if only on a superficial level. We adopt our schools, states, countries, and even professional sports teams in order to feel solidarity with a group. Being alone was a major threat to the survival of our ancestors, and today we, as their descendants, continue to expend large amounts of attention and energy in order to avoid being alone. This should come as no surprise if we look at our human history, since we have lived together in small groups, tribes, or villages for the vast majority of our time on earth.

However, in our frenetic, mobile, youth-oriented society, older adults are placed on the fringes of everyday life and seen as nonessential once their children are grown. To age in our society is to become more isolated: as our child-raising acquaintances move out of our lives, as our offspring move out of the house, as we retire from our work, as our neighbors move to their retirement place, and sadly, as our spouse dies. And with this isolation comes a greater risk for disease-accelerated decline.

We are wired to be together

During my time as a student at the National Defense University in Washington, DC, I was privileged to travel to the then Soviet Union as part of the curriculum. I was there specifically to observe the Soviet medical system, and I was able to visit Moscow, Volgograd (formerly Stalingrad), Tbilisi in Georgia, and Saint Petersburg. During our visit in Moscow, our group toured several large apartment buildings, built during the Khrushchev years, which housed hundreds of people. These buildings had paper-thin walls, and as we walked the hallways, we could hear babies crying, televisions, conversations, music, and dogs barking. When we returned to the bus, I asked the guide how it was possible to live with such noise and lack of privacy. I remember her answer to the word. "In Russia, our winters are long and cold. To hear a human voice on the other side of the wall is comforting." Yes, we are indeed wired that way.

In fact, the natural tendency to form social units and emotional attachment is not unique to humans. Our cerebral cortex, the outermost layer of our brain, is more highly developed than that of all other mammals. This gives us keener capabilities of memory, language, perceptual awareness, thought, and some of the more specialized motor skills. However, the area of the brain just below our cerebral cortex, the limbic or paleomammalian brain, arose, as the name suggests, early in mammals. Despite its early origins, this part of the brain persists today in all mammals. It is responsible, according to famous neuroscientist Paul MacLean, for the motivation and emotion involved in feeding, reproductive, and parental behavior, and therefore for much of our drive for social connection.[2] Even beyond this, it has been hypothesized that even our human capacity for empathy and nonverbal connection, the very basis of social connection, is centered in this area of the brain, which, again, we share with other mammals.[3] This shared capacity is just further evidence of a deep evolutionary basis for our drive for social connection and perhaps part of the explanation for why it's possible for many of us to derive deep emotional attachment and support from our pets.

We are, in fact, herd creatures. If you have ever observed other herd animals, it is clear that their behavior is influenced significantly by being with, or wanting to be with, others. Take horses, for instance. When part of a herd, a horse is more interactive, spirited, and physically active. Alone in a pasture, he is quiet, or, in some cases, anxious. If you introduce any other creature, even a chicken, the horse will "buddy up" with that other beast rather than be alone. We are similarly wired, with a preference for our own species but a definite aversion to being alone. Our penal system knows this all too well. When prisoners are unruly or difficult to manage, solitary confinement is a powerful tool to modify behavior. According to Drs. Toni Antonucci and Bob Kahn, we journey through our lives with a social support network, which they call a "social support convoy" to emphasize that these networks are dynamic, changing with our life situation and our personal development.[4] And it's a good thing that they do change, for removal from some sort of social support network is disorienting, painful, and a powerful stressor.

In a remarkable study published in 2012, bees were the subject of research on social interaction and aging. When bees age, they are removed from the duties of caring for the young and other hive-related tasks. They are assigned the task of foraging (i.e., flying out from the hive to find sources of food and nectar). This study showed rapid deterioration of the brain in these foraging bees. When, however, these bees were experimentally reinserted into the hive to care for the young, their brain deterioration reversed![5]

The new discovery of "mirror neurons" seems to highlight the idea that we are wired for social interaction. When mammals do something and when they observe something being done, the same neurons fire in their brains. Say, for instance, that you see another person in physical distress. You brain responds by activating the areas of your brain that would be activated were you in that same type of physical distress. The same goes for sadness or elation. This mirroring is theorized to have many purposes, from learning to empathy, but the presence of this ability is yet another example of the social wiring of our brains.[6]

Recently, I had to have a tooth extracted. Now, I am a product of a fluoride-ignorant generation that experienced dentistry devoid of movies in the ceiling, colorful scrubs, and painless procedures. And despite decades of technological advances, pulling a tooth still comes down to wrestling an unwilling enamel-coated appendage out of its bone home. Yes, there was novocaine and an explanation of what was about to happen, but the primitive deed still reeked of a scene from *Les Misérables* and brought back memories of dental-office dread. What helped me most, what gave me the most comfort, was the hand of Brona, the surgical assistant, on my shoulder. Whenever she wasn't busy she rested her hand there, and that made everything less threatening, more doable. We are not wired to be isolated creatures, especially in difficult times.

I have seen dying people become more peaceful with this basic empathetic gesture. We are beginning to be able to explain such things in biochemical terms, but that does not in any way negate that we are creatures who derive desirable and salubrious effects from being with others; in fact, it validates this view.

All this is not to say that we don't seek out time alone to reflect, be at peace, or otherwise "recharge our batteries." And life has a way of damaging us, with friends, family, or just another of our own species; people can hurt us in a way that causes us to throw up defensive walls and to be wary of others, and, for the more damaged, to prefer to be alone rather than risk being hurt. Despite this, most of us, most of the time, prefer company.

So, we ask ourselves, can it be that something so deeply rooted in our

brains and therefore in our nature as social connection is not only desirable, important for survival, but also more healthy for us? Once again,
Patsy from Minnesota weighs in: "You betcha." In fact, it appears we are
not healthy humans *unless* we are connected to others of our species. It is
a critical component of our authentic health.

Better together

In his thought-provoking 2000 book *Bowling Alone,* Harvard University
professor of public policy Robert Putnam tracks the decline in Americans' participation in social organizations over the last quarter of the
twentieth century.[7] He concludes that we are paying a significant health
price for that disengagement. He reviews a wealth of research, which
leads him to conclude that the link between social connectedness and
health and well-being is perhaps the most well established of all the
areas of study of social connection.

Longitudinal studies (observational studies that look at the same
variables over a long period) in Alameda and Tecumseh, as well as in
Scandinavia and Japan, have clearly established a relationship between
social connection and health. People who are socially disconnected
or isolated are between two and five times more likely to die from *all
causes* compared to matched individuals who have close ties with family,
friends, and community.[8] And according to these same studies, people
who are connected have more positive health outcomes than those not
so connected. These studies have established beyond reasonable doubt
that social connectedness is one of the most powerful determinants of
our well-being. The more integrated we are with our community, the less
likely we are to experience colds, heart attacks, strokes, cancer, depression, and premature death of all sorts.[9]

Why this is true is not so easy to determine. Social networks may provide necessary resources such as money or transportation, which might
reduce stress. Or, social networks, particularly if they consist of healthy
people, may reinforce healthy behaviors. An even more interesting possibility, however, is that lack of social connection depresses immune
function. The mechanism is thought to be stress, which is more common
with isolation or lack of social support. Within a village environment,
our ancestors were part of the whole; each individual was a small part
of a larger organism with a higher purpose. As the village went, so did

they. In times of trouble, the village was there to help. Today, we function more as individuals with a real and threatening fear that we will have to deal with trouble essentially on our own. Whether it's financial or health-related or work-related problems, we will have to handle it alone. This situation is dramatically different from how we evolved and results in a lingering, ever-present stress—chronic production of the glucocorticoids seen with stress, which, in turn, suppresses immune function. Dr. Janice Kiecolt-Glaser and her colleagues have established a strong relationship between stress, immunological competence, and health.[10] Too much stress, or the chronic stress common in our frenetic society today, leaves the immune system weak or not functioning optimally, and this, in turn, leaves us vulnerable to a variety of diseases, including cardiovascular disease, cancer, depression, and infections.

Moreover, societies today value independence and personal control. We are drawn to the likes of the strong, capable men and women who can "do it all," who know exactly what they want in life, and who go get it. This might be an admired image, but it is one that leaves the individual out there alone doing battle with others in order to succeed. Such a view is understandably highly stressful and frequently engages the fight-or-flight mechanism, since, in fact, success or failure, one's very survival, is seen to be dependent on the individual's actions alone. The village societies of our ancestors—and some communities that existed even as late as the early twentieth century—valued the common good over that of the individual. The ability to work with others to achieve a mutually beneficial goal was highly admired. When adversity struck, it was viewed as a common challenge and significant support was available. When my barn burned down, the village would mobilize and help me rebuild. Consequently there would tend to be less stress, less cortisol, and better immune system function in such societies.

Martin Seligman, a University of Pennsylvania psychologist, wrote in *Psychology Today* years ago about "Boomer Blues." He attributed a pervasive unhappiness in the baby boomers to a generational belief in personal control and autonomy over commitment to duty and common enterprise.[11] I believe he is alluding to the lack of this sense of the common good as both a motivator and a social connector, which our ancestors cultivated out of necessity.

One of my first assignments in the Air Force was at a fighter base in Germany during the Cold War. I was assigned to take care of the flyers and families of the 53rd Tactical Fighter Squadron and I was their flight surgeon. They adopted me and welcomed me as a fellow aviator, even writing my name on one of the F15s. I flew with Bubba and Fonz and Bush (the tactical call signs of Mike, Rick, and Dave) and others. I deployed with them. Paula and I traveled and partied with their families. We mourned the loss of our comrades as a community. And we all felt the profound sense of both camaraderie and a higher purpose in our lives. I confess I have never felt the same level of satisfaction as I experienced with the 53rd TFS. And I'm not alone. Our periodic squadron reunions are big events in our lives. We witness together the weddings of our children. Years, even decades, fade away when we meet. We are forever bonded: a band of brothers, rarely found today, but the necessary rule for our distant ancestors. My deep sense of satisfaction stems from the fact that we as a species have a strong predilection for such bands, but they are getting more difficult to find.

I have a friend, Fred, who lives in a small town in Kansas. In addition to his day job, he serves as the editor of the local newspaper, published only four times per year. Fred sends me the *Tipton Times*, and in those few pages I follow the lives of the town's several hundred residents: births, deaths, graduations, athletic accomplishments, accidents, agricultural reports, store openings and closures, the return of the railroad, the school plays, the dance recitals. I follow the lives of those who move away from Tipton, as they go to college, work, and even die in another place. And somewhere along the way I began to care. I evolved from reading Fred's paper with bemusement to nostalgia. I, in fact, grew up in a larger town, but as a child, my world was small. I can easily substitute names from my old neighborhood for these Tipton names. And I believe the nostalgia goes even deeper, to some place within me that was handed down to me by many ancestors over eons—a sense of my humanity related to place and, more importantly, related to others. There is some of Tipton in all of us, and we need it to be healthy.

Blue Zones rule, and Roseto is rosy

We see other examples of these village-like societies today. Earlier in this book we discussed Blue Zones, areas where extreme longevity is much more common than in other societies. In areas of Okinawa, Sardinia, Costa Rica, and Greece, there are common characteristics of those who live long. Two of those characteristics are (1) family is put ahead of other concerns, and (2) people of all ages are socially active and integrated into their communities.

In *Bowling Alone*, Dr. Robert Putnam describes a well-studied town in Pennsylvania that clearly illustrated the effects of social connection on health. Roseto, Pennsylvania, was also mentioned in Malcolm Gladwell's book *Outliers*, because of the virtual absence of heart disease in the town, even in the mid-twentieth century, when the nation as a whole and even neighboring towns were experiencing rising incidences of heart attacks. The town was the focus of long-term studies that ultimately established stress as a major cause of heart disease. So why was there less stress in Roseto?

The small town of approximately 1,500 people had been founded and populated by immigrants from the same region in Italy. Strong community resources, such as a mutual-aid society, churches, athletic fields, and sports clubs, together with a value system that scorned displays of wealth and encouraged tight social connection, were the distinguishing features. Rosetans drew on one another for emotional and financial support, frequently congregating on front porches or in clubs. And when the new generation of adults arrived in the 1980s and this socially mobile group began to reject some of the old ways of their parents and grandparents, the protection against heart disease began to fade.

Regardless of the mechanism, an excellent comprehensive review of the literature on social connectedness and health led by Julianne Holt-Lunstad from Brigham Young University concluded that "strong social relationships influence the health outcomes of adults," with 50 percent more likelihood of longevity, whereas "social isolation is the risk equivalent of smoking for heart disease and cancer."[12]

Although we cannot go back to the village environments of our ancestors, if we understand the importance of social connection and work to make it a core element of our modern-day environments, perhaps we can find authentic health and indeed reap the health rewards of our ancestors.

Better than ever?

So, questions then arise: Aren't we more connected than ever? With Facebook, cell phones, emails, texts, and tweets, don't we have more "friends"? Aren't we "talking" to more people every day? Shouldn't we be getting healthier? As these are relatively new technologies, it remains to be demonstrated whether this will happen. However, if we use our ancestors as a guide to what specifically we need from being connected to others, we can make some guesses.

It's true we need to communicate with others as a basic way to connect. It has been estimated that as much as two-thirds of communication is nonverbal:[13] gestures, body position, facial features, and eye contact, for example. This would make us question whether some of these technologies deliver on promises to enhance communication. Certainly they would seem to act as "connectors" in that they have the capacity to bring people together physically, as seen in social media–driven actions like Occupy Wall Street and the Libyan uprisings.

The most salubrious effects of social connection are seen when we have at least a small number of very close friends, people we would have no reluctance to call at 3:00 a.m. if necessary. Unfortunately, we seem to be going in the opposite direction from this more beneficial social culture. According to a study in the *American Sociological Review*, Americans are thought to be suffering a loss in the quality and quantity of close friendships since at least 1985. The study states that 25 percent of Americans have no close confidants and that the average total number of confidants per person has dropped from four to two.[14]

Some of the beneficial effects of social interaction require touching, as with babies. The financial and emotional support systems seen in Roseto might be possible from a distance, but the frequent meetings, club environments, and sharing of narrated stories might not be. So, it would seem that our modern technologies for social networking have wider reach, the potential to bring people together physically, and the ability to "keep in touch." However, as with other beneficial effects based in our evolutionary biology, it would seem the face-to-face, rubbing elbows–type social interaction of our ancestors is most likely more associated with the powerful health benefits of social engagement.

My good friend Erich, who lives in Bavaria, believes it is better to communicate in person and that, if you cannot, then sending letters is the best substitute. He is not alone, but this cadre of traditional communicators is on the wane. Will we, like the new generation in Roseto, begin to lose the health effects of social connection? More studies will be necessary to determine the health value of our social networking technologies. In her provocative book, *Alone Together*, Sherry Turkle, professor of the social studies of science and technology at MIT, tells of the "gathering clouds" presented by technology in relation to our absolutely critical social relations: "On social networks, people are reduced to their profiles. On our mobile devices, we often talk to each other on the move and with little disposable time—so little, in fact, that we communicate in a new language of abbreviations in which letters stand for words and emotions for feelings. We don't ask the open ended 'How are you?' Instead we ask the more limited 'Where are you?' and 'What's up?' These are good questions for getting someone's location and making a simple plan. They are not good for opening a dialogue about complexity of feeling. We are increasingly connected to each other but oddly more alone."[15] Albert Einstein was more direct. "I fear the day that technology surpasses human interaction. The world will have a generation of idiots."

Ethel and her magnificent rose-colored glasses

She is ninety years old, is a caretaker for her progressively more forgetful husband, has been widowed twice, and is a recent cancer survivor. Yet Ethel, a former Ms. New York Senior America, continues to reach out to people. She has skills: performing, singing, dancing, even comedic skills; writing and teaching skills; and people skills. She uses all these to stay engaged, to give meaning and purpose to her life, and to bring happiness to those around her.

Ethel lives in a Masterpiece Living retirement community in South Florida. Despite her recent challenges, she has cajoled, coached, and motivated her neighbors, most of whom have never performed in any capacity, to step out of their isolation and reluctance—and step high— in a Broadway-style show that Ethel directs. Ethel has transformed her amateur performers; has made them proud of themselves; has made them more engaged in life, some more than when they were decades younger. She has created a social network of performers and audience members so powerful that the entire community has been transformed into a vital and flourishing place to continue to grow.

Still writing a column for a New York publication targeted to older adults, and still involved with the Ms. New York Senior America pageant that she headed for decades, Ethel is tireless. She has performed at the White House, had her own radio show, taught exercise for decades, written an autobiography, and has basically swallowed life whole. And even as we speak together, she breaks into an original song about her community and about Masterpiece Living. To the tune of "Oklahoma":

> La Posada we will laugh and sing and even dance.
> And who knows what may come if you meet someone.
> There may even be a new romance.
> We're so happy that we are all here.
> Let's stand up and give a loud, lusty, cheer.

Ethel remains a brilliant force of vitality and resilience, still looking glamorous and younger than her years, but mostly she is out on the playing field of life. Always with others, connected by song, and dance, and comedy. Always helping others to reach beyond their comfort zone and marvel at the result. Ethel is a life coach, a meteoric blaze of benevolent light for all who meet her. She knows the secret of social connection and shares that secret with everyone she meets. She could easily have chosen to wallow in her life's turn of events, but instead she chose life. Ernest Hemingway wrote in *A Farewell to Arms*, "The world breaks everyone and afterward many are strong in the broken places." Ethel is people strong.

❦ Masterpiece Living Pearls for Staying Connected

1. We're back in the easy chair again, thinking. How many people do you see in a day? A week? Do you know anyone that you could call at 3:00 a.m. for help? Are there people in your life who would be comfortable calling you at 3:00 a.m.? Relative to your association with other people, how do you want the rest of your life to be? Who do you want in it? Do you welcome people into your life or keep them at a distance? These questions, like the Lifestyle Inventory you took in chapter 4, provide a snapshot of where you are relative to where you want to be.

2. Let's get more specific. Who stimulates and energizes you? Who makes you feel better about yourself and the world? Who makes you feel like you could do almost anything? Who was meaningful in your life and is now absent?

These are the people you want to nurture. Like plants, friendships need attention, nourishment, and effort to keep them from
fading from your life, and to allow them to grow. Yes, social connections require work, and who has the time, right? You do. It's
a matter of priorities. We cannot expect that friends will be there
when we finally have the time or inclination to connect again if we
don't nourish them, if we are not the kind of person they prefer to
be with. How to nourish? It's simply a matter of communicating
with them, of letting them know they are important in your life.
Whatever it takes.

3. Have you decided that there are too few people in your life? How
can you grow the number of people with whom you are connected
in some way? Like dating, getting to know people can take a lot of
work, and sometimes you find in the end that you have little in common. If this happens repeatedly, it is easy to become disillusioned
and to give up trying altogether. So go back to question #1 and think
about what you want your life to be in this next phase. What sort of
things do you want to be doing? Well, just like in Tip One, these are
the things you should be doing. *Do the things you love; the people
will follow.* And the people who do will most likely be people with
whom you have a lot in common. If you enjoy learning, take a class.
Bicycling? Get on that bike, and maybe join a bicycling club. Writing? Find a writer's group. Gardening? You get it, right?

4. Social networking resources can help you locate and connect with
significant people who have disappeared from your life. More than
likely they will be very happy to hear from you and want to meet.
What do you have to lose?

5. What about people who drain you? Who make you feel bad about
yourself? Who are not happy when you have a success or other positive event in your life? We are responsible for our internal environment, and if that's negative, for whatever reason, we will be negative
and we will be raising our risk for disease. So, it's time to purge those
negative elements. It doesn't have to be a big scene. No drama, only
stop connecting with them, or if necessary, respectfully tell them
how you feel and that you want to move on. Wish them luck. You
may even want to give them a rain check for when they become
more positive, but more than likely that will only delay the inev-

itable. Make it a clean break and make room for the new people who will nourish you and whom you will nourish in return. When I left the military, I reached out to neighbors and coworkers in my new town. This town was, however, a place that people rarely left and so the lives of its inhabitants were filled with family and friends they had gone to kindergarten with. This was fine for them, but it left them no room, in their minds, for new friends—bad for me. So clean out your social closet and make the room. It will be an adventure well worth the effort.

TIP 5

LOWER YOUR RISKS

We are what we repeatedly do. Excellence, then,
is not an act but a habit.
—ARISTOTLE

ost think that one day, perhaps when we least expect it, fate comes knocking on our door and there it is: cancer, or heart disease, or dementia, or whatever else we fear most. Although such a scenario can be terrifying, in some ways it's comforting. Why? Because if that is indeed how we get sick, then there's not much we can do about it, is there? It's fate. We're going to get it or we're not. This is, in fact, the rationale many use to justify dangerous behavior, like smoking or overeating. "You've got to die of something, right?" or "Hey, I'll get it or I won't, I'm not going to worry about it." Or the famous "I know a guy who lived to be a hundred . . ."

Of course, when we were ignorant of the mechanisms and causes of disease, these arguments held some water. Now, however, we know that how we age, and therefore what diseases knock on our door, is dependent primarily on our lifestyle. In fact, 50 percent to 75 percent of US cancer deaths are caused by three harmful behaviors: tobacco use, lack of exercise, and poor diet.[1] Even higher percentages of coronary heart disease and stroke are considered to be preventable with lifestyle and preventive measures. The slowing of the progression of dementia, the delay of its onset, and perhaps even prevention of it are beginning to look possible (see Tip Three). Yes, the argument that fate will have its way and that we are totally helpless is beginning to show some serious leaks.

Each of us has risks for disease or injury. These risks arise from our life experiences, lifestyle choices, and, to a lesser extent, genes. I believe many risks arise when we live a lifestyle far removed from our core needs. What is becoming clearer with recent research is that these risks are, for the most part, manageable. Actually, better than manageable—we can reduce or even eliminate many risks altogether.

What you don't know *will* hurt you

We are conditioned, perhaps by our youthful way of learning, or by the piecemeal way that research on health is revealed to us, to think of life-style and health in linear terms—that is, if I do this, this will happen. If I exercise regularly, I will lose weight, look better, get fit, and decrease the chances of a heart attack. If I stop smoking, I'll reduce my chances of lung cancer. If I get regular checkups, I'll be less likely to get cancer. If I eat right, I'll lose weight and not get diabetes or have a stroke or heart attack. If I do crossword puzzles, I'll keep my brain sharp. Our approach to lifestyle is piecemeal, fractionated like our medical approach to disease, and we think of skin ailments, heart ailments, neurological diseases, or gastrointestinal diseases, not a sick *person*. And even more common reasons for making lifestyle changes, such as increasing physical activity, frequently have little to do with avoiding disease and more to do with looking better.

When we are younger, we frequently attempt to adopt healthier lifestyles for non-health reasons. Vanity is perhaps the major driver of physical activity in the young. Being more attractive, looking better at that wedding or on the beach, is a strong motivator. Competitive advantage in sports or bragging-rights accomplishments are very common in males, and becoming more so in women.

The problems with these more simplistic motivators toward healthy lifestyles is that once we are beyond them in our lives, when sexual attraction or bragging rights are less powerful as reasons to undertake change, what then happens? Frequently, we are less likely to attempt change at all. We consider that growth and positive changes are things of the past and become accepting of the way things are.

Making changes for a particular beneficial outcome can be effective.

For example, attempting to ward off heart disease, particularly if we have a family history, or a specific risk factor, makes sense. Even when the reason is superficial, such as vanity, these efforts can help people accomplish great things. Sometimes, even when the vanity fades, basic fear of getting old, or breaking a hip and losing independence, can be a powerful motivator with older adults. But the approaches that focus on a very specific and tangible outcome, in my opinion, miss a fundamental reality of managing our risk, and actually limit what we can achieve with lifestyle modification.

The warrior in us

Being alive renders all of us at risk for disease, injury, and early death. But once again, it is not that fate one day decides to knock on your door and in comes heart disease or cancer or dementia. These threats are always with us by virtue of our having a pulse. It is as if risks are like buzzards orbiting above us waiting for an opportunity. Yes, for some unfortunates, they strike serendipitously, without regard for age or lifestyle. But for the majority of us, it is we who unintentionally open our doors to them.

The Art of War is a series of essays written over 2,400 years ago by Chinese military strategist Sun Tzu. Although, as the title suggests, it is about the conduct of war, it has been a reference for many on how to conduct themselves in business, sports, or any competitive endeavor, and tucked within its pages on military strategy are gems for managing risk, including this one:

> It is a doctrine of war not to assume the enemy will not come, but rather to rely on one's readiness to meet him; not to presume that he will not attack, but rather to make oneself invincible.[2]

Making ourselves "invincible" against disease, is that possible? No, not completely invincible, but the research on aging and the lifestyle contribution to disease would indicate that we can go a long way in preventing disease or injury, or at least become more resistant. So, maybe the warrior analogy is a good one. In fact, many view staying healthy as a struggle, a competition against multiple threats to a healthy state. Rather than think in linear terms (i.e., doing one thing in order to prevent another), we should think in whole-body terms. Approaching our risks in this way forces us to address our basic core requirements for health, those we have in common with our ancestors, those authentic needs.

So, how do we keep our whole selves strong, resilient, and resistant to all threats? Should we be like the warrior who keeps himself strong, not just physically but mentally, emotionally, and spiritually, and who is therefore ready to defend himself against any threat? The warrior who doesn't "assume the enemy will not come," but who in fact assumes that if he is not as strong as he can be, the enemy will come? This whole-person approach to defending oneself against disease threats is exactly what this book is about. The Ten Tips are in fact a training program for the health warrior, a way to keep oneself as invincible as possible. Not so much targeting any one disease, but *all threats*. It is a training program to develop a lifestyle that defends and strengthens our core needs: a training program in authentic health.

By keeping our bodies moving, we prevent falls, strengthen our heart, lower blood sugar, keep our mind sharp, strengthen our immune defenses, lower the chance for osteoporosis, have a more positive attitude, and more. By staying socially connected, our immune system functions better and we resist disease and recover more quickly when we do get sick. By laughing, we enhance our immune defenses and are more likely to stay engaged. Having a solid purpose will sustain us through lean and challenging times. And on and on. These lifestyle strategies are intricately interrelated, just like all our body systems. Strengthening one area affects others and builds a stronger, more robust, more invincible whole.

And there's more to being invincible. The good warrior also understands that he must know his enemy. He must know where he is at risk of being overpowered. And he knows that when in battle, he must depend on comrades in order to triumph. So, too, when the enemy is disease. If we are to win against disease and impairment, we not only must be strong; we must also know our risk, and attack that risk. Reliable comrades in that battle are those who are committed to making and keeping us healthy and who know the enemy well. These comrades-in-arms are the health professionals available to us. To ignore them, to avoid them or the help they offer us, is both foolish and risky.

And as with most things, there is a potential dark side to our comrades. Recent research indicates that risks for unhealthy conditions or disease tend to occur in clusters.[3] These findings tell us that risky lifestyle factors, such as obesity or smoking or a sedentary lifestyle, often are a common characteristic of certain groups. Basically, we can draw one of two conclusions from this research: We associate with people who have lifestyles like our own, or we tend to adopt the lifestyle of those with whom we associate—along with the risks that come with it. The take-away? Associate with people who have healthy lifestyles.

Two big players in our quest for resilience

We have been discussing the fact that it is a whole-person approach to lifestyle that lowers risk and builds the resilience that leads to authentic health and successful aging. Two areas in particular relate to this approach and therefore deserve more discussion: stress and nutrition.

Stress: The Big Uneasy

Most assume that the threats to our health and aging are in the environment around us. Yet one of the most deadly and pervasive enemies, like a Trojan horse, is potentially within each of us. As I have done a couple of times already in this book, I'm going to call stress "the Big Uneasy," because this accurately represents its effects on us. The concept of stress and even the word itself is overused, poorly understood, and means different things to different people. In our achievement-oriented world, there are many strongly held yet unsubstantiated views about the relationship between stress and health and aging. How can we accomplish anything unless we challenge ourselves (read as "stress" ourselves)? Don't we have to push ourselves beyond our comfort level to succeed? And even if we're not in a dog-eat-dog competitive world, life has a way of bringing lots of "stuff" that "stresses us out." Many believe that stress is necessary to stimulate our bodies and minds in order to be stronger; they see stress as providing us with a boot camp–type challenge so that we become more resilient.

So, we ask ourselves, is stress good or bad? Does it help us or hurt us? How does a whole-person, warrior approach to lifestyle relate to the stress in our lives? Does stress really cause disease?

Dr. Robert Sapolsky, professor of biological sciences at Stanford, in his foreword to Bruce McEwen's brilliant book on stress and stress-related disease, *The End of Stress As We Know It*, underlines the importance of this holistic lifestyle approach:

> We've entered the gilded genomics era just in time to have
> to admit that most of our ills have to do with extraordinarily

ungenomic things like your psychological makeup and patterns of social relations, your social status and the society
in which you have that status, your lifestyle. And at the center of this nexus is stress—what stressors we are exposed to
and how we cope. Most of us will live long enough and well
enough to get seriously ill with a stress-related disease.[4]

Is Sapolsky telling us that that in addition to our lifestyle, stress
can weaken our defenses? That stress, the Big Uneasy, that seemingly
ever-present characteristic of modern life, can raise our risk of, and even
perhaps bring on, disease?

The answer is a resounding yes, and Dr. McEwen, head of the neuro-
endocrinology lab at Rockefeller University in New York City, gives us
a remarkably clear explanation of the mechanism of what some call the
scourge of modern man in his excellent book.[5]

According to McEwen, all mammals developed in an environment
rich in potential threats to their existence. It was necessary for survival,
then, to be able to respond to those threats. There were threats targeting
the internal state, such as environmentally caused changes in body temperature, the oxygen saturation of blood, or blood pressure. These threats
were managed automatically by mechanisms that evolved to maintain a
fairly steady internal state called homeostasis.

McEwen prefers the broader, newer term *allostasis* to describe the
stable state provided by systems able to change with the requirements
placed on them. Threats to mammals' very lives, such as predators,
required an intricate, variable, and immediate response, which basically
provided the energy to fight or flee. This fight-or-flight response is common to all mammals and involves powerful "do or die" settings within
many of our body's systems. For many mammals, however, particularly humans, the threat environment has changed. As McEwen notes,
"It seems that allostasis has not caught up with evolution and is not yet
convinced that such dramatic physical responses are becoming less necessary." So, he notes further, "a council member standing up at a town
meeting, or a violinist stepping before the audience, may feel they are
gearing up, involuntarily, to vanquish their opponent or propel themselves away." We've all felt this. It's the stuff of heroic stories of rescuers
lifting cars off trapped people, but also of the pounding pulse, tremors,
and rapid breathing associated with a job interview.

And there's the rub. We humans are, as far as we know, the only
mammal capable of *self-inducing* this fight-or-flight mechanism, and its

all-systems-go response, *with our thoughts*! Moreover, we seem to be the only mammal capable of *sustaining* a chronic state of hyper-response—our brains being the primary engine behind this—even when there is no immediate or even real threat. This type of stress McEwen calls "allostatic load." "It usually seems to kick in when we don't want it to," he says. "Increasingly, the situations that ignite the stress response are ones for which neither fight or flight is an option—working for an overbearing boss, for example. . . . And so, deprived of its natural result, the very system designed to protect us begins to cause wear and tear instead, and illness sets in."[6]

And indeed the list of illnesses and conditions related to chronic stress is impressive because the adverse effects of chronic stress involve the cardiovascular system, the brain, and the immune system itself. Sheldon Cohen, a Carnegie Mellon psychologist, writes, "Effects of stress on regulation of immune and inflammatory processes have the potential to influence depression, infectious, autoimmune, and coronary artery disease, and at least some (e.g., viral) cancers."[7]

In fact, there are many who believe that stress has the potential to be a factor in the progression, if not the cause, of a virtual Who's Who of ailments, from the common cold to ulcers to dementia. We see, then, that our internal protection system against threats, in an environment where stress is more common, as in our frenetic, multitasking, hard-charging, and noisy world, begins to cause us harm.

And how does Dr. McEwen propose we handle this stress so that we don't become "stressed out"? You guessed it—with our lifestyle choices. Once again, the recommendations included in these Ten Tips offer opportunities to manage this allostatic load to a point where we can avoid the harm or at least minimize it. Yes, those things we heard about for so long—physical movement, social connection, adequate sleep, eating well—these turn out to be major players in our efforts to not only look and feel good but also to control our uniquely human response to stress so that it does not run awry and work against us. The warrior within us, in fact, must be, ironically, watchful of our self-induced threats.

Nutrition: Fueling the Engine of Health and Successful Aging

The second major lifestyle characteristic I would like to focus on in order to lower our risks is nutrition. Although the Ten Tips are pretty comprehensive, eating right did not make the top ten primary topics, but not because I don't consider nutrition essential to good health and successful aging. On the contrary, I consider it to be an essential part of healthy aging and therefore decided to make it a key point in this discussion of lowering our risk for disease and impairment. I cannot hope to be comprehensive in my comments on eating as it applies to lifestyle and successful aging. There are bookshelves filled with solid information on the topic, and I am humble enough to not attempt to duplicate such erudite works. Instead, I would like to address some important considerations for aging in a better way that are rarely discussed in such works (at least not as primary considerations).

For decades now in the United States, the discourse regarding eating has been dominated by a fixation on weight, much like the focus on exercise. The term *diet*, in fact, is today synonymous with "weight-loss program," even though the word derives from Greek and meant "a manner of living." In our culture, the word usually refers to a manipulation of our food intake in order to achieve weight loss rather than to the entirety of *what* we eat. Nutrition, on the other hand, the more important consideration of providing our bodies the food necessary to support life, gets lost in the rhetoric and sensationalism of weight loss. It's not that addressing the rampant problem of obesity is not important. Obesity is associated with multiple serious threats to our health, independence, and even our very lives: cardiovascular disease, cancer, diabetes, and dementia. A 2002 RAND research brief noted that obesity, in fact, poses more of a threat for having multiple chronic conditions than smoking or heavy drinking of alcohol.[8]

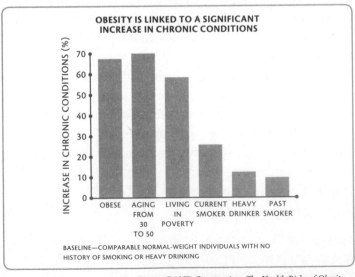

Source: RAND Corporation, *The Health Risks of Obesity*.

It is nutrition, however, that is the overarching concern here, for it encompasses situations of dietary imbalance, like obesity, and even more importantly, the nourishment necessary to enable us to perform at our best, to be resilient, and to ward off threats to our health. Our core needs are about nourishment. Our approach to authentic health is not about deprivation, but about providing for our core nutritional needs.

For most of the time that man and his immediate primate ancestors have inhabited the earth, he ate the foods that provided the most energy for the least amount of physical energy expended—i.e., foods that were readily available. Therefore, the diet of our ancestors consisted mostly of fruits, wild vegetables, nuts, fish, and small amounts of meat (plus and including beans, flowers, gums, fungi, stems, shellfish, eggs, small mammals, fish, frogs, turtles, and other similar available foods). These foods had less available energy (calories) per gram and more vitamins, minerals, amino acids, and fiber than foods we eat today. Sugar, other than what naturally occurred in the foods they foraged, did not exist. Since sophisticated hunting implements and domesticated animals are relatively new phenomena in our history, meat was available primarily from small animals or as remnants from predator kills. In either case, game animals would have been less fatty than our modern-day animals, and what fat there was would have been less saturated.[9] It is not a leap, therefore, to propose that human physiology—which evolved during this period that constitutes a vast majority of the time we have walked the earth—requires these types of food in order to function at its best. Hence the USDA nutritional recommendation to eat at least five help-ings of fruits and vegetables daily. The recent resurgence of interest in the Paleo diet is based on the belief that we do indeed require foods eaten by our distant ancestors to be healthy.

Basically, because our ancestors had limited access to food and because survival was on the line, they would readily eat high-calorie food, like fats, whenever they encountered it, which was hardly ever. They were, and we are, "wired" to eat high-calorie food whenever it's available. And so it is also not difficult to understand the modern-day plague of obesity when we now have ready access to food much higher in caloric content and from sources our bodies are not designed to deal with. Foods with ele-ments unknown to our ancestors, such as trans fats (found in some chips, crackers, and pastries), simple carbohydrates (soda, candy, and pastries are abundant sources), and added sugar, compound the problem.

Such food, rare to our ancestors, is not only available every hundred yards in some cities but is also very inexpensive. In fact, this is the first time in human history that the poorer populations (at least in the United States and other developed countries) are overweight rather than thin. Fast food is cheaper and high in fat and calories. So, large segments of the population continue this pattern of eating what gives the highest energy content for the least amount of physical effort. Additionally, our modern cultural custom of eating at three prescribed times of day is dramatically different from that of our ancestors, who ate frequent small meals depending on availability. Those meals were ridiculously small compared to today's supersized ones. So not only the quality of our food, but also the quantity, differs greatly from that which guided the evolution of our physiology.

Last, physical movement was an absolute requirement of the daily activities of our ancestors. Therefore the expenditure of calories was not something done in one's spare time but a nonnegotiable necessity.

So, do we have to wonder why we are obese? Why we are plagued by cardiovascular diseases, cancer, dementia, and diabetes? We have departed greatly from the foods, eating patterns, and activity level that determined our current physiology. Evolution is a much slower process than cultural change and the development of high-calorie fast food. It's not that we must return to our ancestral diets, but we can use them as a general guide. Eating smaller portions, more often, perhaps six times daily, with fruits, vegetables, nuts, and beans being the core of our diet—this alone can serve as a huge step forward to lowering health risks, enhancing our nutrition, and achieving authentic health.

Aristotle said life isn't worth living without chocolate. Actually, he didn't, but he did say "All things in moderation," and those are words to abide by if you want to live well, and age well. We should mix it up and sample carbohydrates, proteins, fats, but do it more judiciously. Realizing that thirst is a late sign of dehydration and that dehydration raises risk of clots, strokes, and heart attacks, we should commit to keep ahead of dehydration with enough non-caffeinated, nonalcoholic beverages. (Aristotle would have undoubtedly approved of alcohol and caffeine—again, in moderation.) So remember to drink water-based drinks *before* you're thirsty.

The United States Department of Agriculture (USDA) has for over one hundred years issued nutrition guidelines. These dietary recommendations, like our knowledge of what constitutes healthy eating, have evolved over that century. For the last twenty years, the USDA's guidance has been in the form of a food pyramid, and the most recent, MyPyramid, was unveiled in 2005 and looked like this:

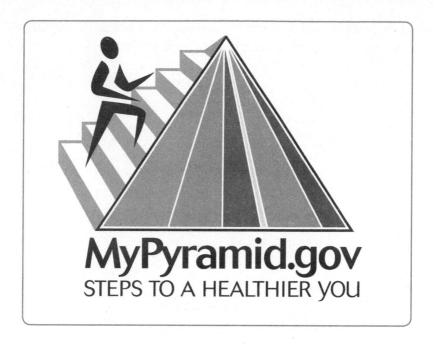

It was then customized for older adults as MyPyramid for Older Adults:

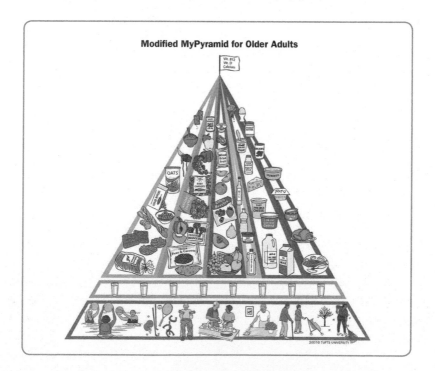

Because these pyramids were thought to be too abstract, in June of 2011 the guidance changed forms and became MyPlate:

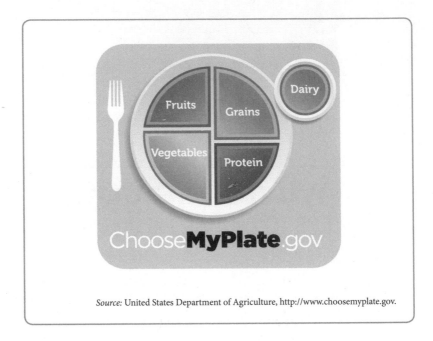

Source: United States Department of Agriculture, http://www.choosemyplate.gov.

MyPlate was intended to be simpler and basically recommended that our diet consist of 30 percent vegetables, 30 percent grains, 20 percent fruits, and 20 percent protein, with a small circle indicating dairy. Additional guidelines are:

- "Make half your plate fruits and vegetables."
- "Switch to skim or 1% milk."
- "Make at least half your grains whole."
- "Vary your protein food choices."

The guidelines also recommend portion control while still enjoying food, as well as reductions in sodium and sugar intake.[10]

In November of 2011, these guidelines were customized for older people by the Jean Mayer USDA Human Nutrition Research Center on Aging at Tufts University, and the result was MyPlate for Older Adults.

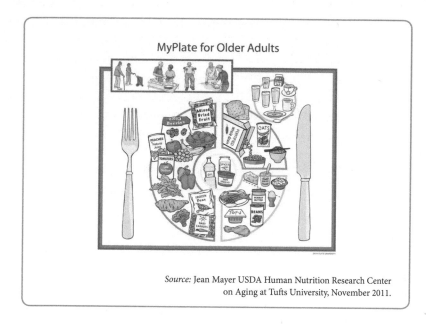

MyPlate for Older Adults

Source: Jean Mayer USDA Human Nutrition Research Center
on Aging at Tufts University, November 2011.

MyPlate for Older Adults focuses on the unique nutritional and physical-activity needs associated with aging and is intended to be a guide for healthy older adults who are living independently and looking for examples of good food choices and physical activities. By emphasizing the consumption of fruits, vegetables, whole grains, and multiple protein sources beyond just meat, as well as the need for physical movement, MyPlate for Older Adults is a close cousin to the diets of our hunter-gatherer and, to some extent, agrarian ancestors. No surprises there, since, as we have stated so strongly in part I of this book, our nutritional and health needs were, we believe, established during the eons of time that predated most of our history as a species and constitute our absolute basic, or authentic, requirements.

Tipping the odds in your favor

We have so much information today that suffering from preventable diseases is all the more tragic. We have learned much about raising our odds against diseases that formerly left us powerless. Take colon cancer. I'm at higher risk since my father had colon cancer. Yet with so much more knowledge about what foods raise or lower the risk of developing it, and with the newer tools for early detection and effective treatment against this disease, which is itself a slow grower, the odds are now hugely in my favor against dying of it . . . as long as I learn all I can about colon cancer, eat better, work with my doctor, and get the recommended screening. And it's the same with so many diseases that are responsible for lower quality—and quantity—of life. So, getting those regular physical exams, the screening tests and immunizations, in addition to making the lifestyle shifts recommended in these Ten Tips, can indeed begin to stack the deck in your favor.

Resilient Mary

Mary knows that if you're truly living, some of life's hits are unavoidable; what is avoidable, however, is having those hits become the beginning of your end. She is ninety-one by the calendar, but at least a decade younger to the eye and all who observe her seize each day. Mary confesses she was treated like a princess as a child and often wonders how she was able to weather the loss of three husbands and significant financial challenges in her earlier life. And not only to weather, but to continue to thrive. Sitting with her as she tells her story, I have no doubt of the source of her indomitable resilience. She has continued to grow even as she enters her tenth decade of life.

"We have lots of parts and all these parts need to be nurtured." Still driving, Mary is not a prisoner of her apartment. She is, rather, frequently spotted, actively engaged within the retirement community where she lives, meeting with people who are considering moving in. "I love meeting and greeting people." Or bringing her signature chicken soup to a neighbor who's ill. Or meeting with the community finance committee. This is right in line with how she lived her life when she was "younger." After "retiring," she volunteered at her city's conference center for over fifteen years, in order to "to be with people." She tells me, "Even if you have quite different ideas on things, you can still connect and have a meaningful relationship." She admits not being an intellectual, but reads to keep on the news of the world and "tries to make sense of life," "taking the good parts of religion to find strength, hope, peace, and spiritual connection." She recently discovered that a local school was in need of teaching assistants and will pursue that possibility. Mary understandably has a soft spot for widows and does all she can to support new widows in her community.

When asked at the conclusion of our interview what advice she would give for aging successfully, she is more forthcoming. "Don't worry about what may happen. Take each day a time. Do something that makes a difference. Be mindful of what others are experiencing." Optimism, purposeful living, and compassion, this is Mary's formula for lowering her own risks and for aging successfully.

Masterpiece Living Pearls for Lowering Your Risks

1. *Find out what your personal risks are.* Use the Lifestyle Inventory to assess your risks. Seek out a health-risk appraisal (there are many available online and from medical insurance companies) for a more comprehensive evaluation. Consult with your physician to get a full understanding of where you are at risk and what she recommends.

2. Using chapter 3, make a plan for *small changes* in order to lower risk. *Do not attempt to address all risks at once.* Seek small, incremental, single changes in order to lower risk. For instance, if you're overweight, begin by eating 10 percent less of your favorite food. When that is a new standard, consider further reducing the amount or adding a second favorite food to reduce incrementally. Or, if you're not eating enough fruits, vegetables, or nuts, add just one helping of one of them that you like each day. The ultimate goal is eating less, eating better foods, and increasing activity, but give yourself as long as it takes to keep moving in a positive direction toward those goals. *Be patient, be kind, be positive.*

3. If the description of "stressed out" fits you, read Tip Seven for more understanding of why you are stressed and what you might do about it. As I write this, I am sitting in a garden in Sedona, Arizona, a very spiritually energizing place for me. I could be out looking for a new restaurant to brag about. I could be out looking for a new trail to hike. I could be worrying about my friends with cancer. But I can also choose to be energized by this garden. To be here alone with the cactus, with the birds singing, with the breeze wafting over my skin, and *not* with my "problems" or my to-do list. I am here in this moment, and it is joyful. Realize that it's not life that is stressing you out—it's your response or interpretation of the never-ending parade of life situations you encounter that is stressing you out. You are the problem. You are the answer!

4. Schedule two or three days to pay careful attention to your eating: what you eat, when you eat, how much you eat, what you are feeling or thinking when you eat. Take a few notes. Now set aside an hour to sit down, read your notes, and make some decisions on what you would like to change. Make sure you are clear on exactly what you want to achieve. Do you want to be thinner? Do you want more energy? Do you want to lower your risk of cancer? Or heart attack? Do you want to live longer? With that outcome in mind, decide on your first step. Don't get too ambitious! For example, say you want to have less knee pain. You should lose some weight. You think you eat too much dessert. So, you might make a plan to leave one small bit of your dessert on your plate. Then you might leave a little more. Next, you might decide to not eat a dessert on one day per week. On that day, do something you enjoy right after eating instead of eating that dessert. Play with your dog; do your hobby; call the grandkids—anything. The rest of your plan will become clear as you see and feel proud of your success with each small step. If you don't accomplish what you'd planned for that day, *do not give up!* You're still better than where you were before, so reboot, redo, or just get back on track. *Guilt and surrender are your enemies*, as are goals that are too ambitious. Do not allow them in your head. You are a warrior, and you can do this.

5. Make sure you partner with a medical practitioner who believes strongly in prevention. You'll know her when she takes time, or has someone on her team take time, to educate you on your risks and risk-lowering strategies. You'll know her when she never gives up on finding ways to *prevent* as well as treat conditions. If you ever hear "Well, you're getting older now, what do you expect?" it's time to move on to another medical practitioner, one who will coach you to lower risk and prevent disease. That, I believe, should be a physician's first role—even before treating and curing disease.

6. Seek out friends who live healthy lifestyles, or at least the lifestyle you are seeking. Whether they intend to or not, they will share it with you. Just as your mother told you, don't hang out with the wrong crowd. Remember that motivational speaker Jim Rohn tell us, "You are the average of the five people you spend the most time with."

NEVER "ACT YOUR AGE"

I'm much too young to be this damn old.
—GARTH BROOKS

I'm not old. I was just born a long time ago.
—JOHN BLOSSOM, AGE NINETY-TWO

How old would you be,
if you didn't know how old you were?
—SATCHEL PAIGE

Men do not quit playing because they grow old;
they grow old because they quit playing.
—OLIVER WENDELL HOLMES

Expectations kill joy. You've experienced this. You're going to lose twenty pounds before the wedding. You lose ten. You're disappointed. Your sister is coming to visit. At last you can resolve all those bad feelings. You have some initial warm moments together but the old resentments come up after only a few hours. You're off to Hawaii for seven days of sun, surf, and relaxation. It rains two days and is cloudy another. Bummer. Yes, we have a penchant for setting expectations high and then lamenting when they don't happen. We can also, however, set expectations too low. Out of ignorance of what's possible, fear of failure, or an attempt to conform to the misguided expectations of family, friends, or peer group, we can sell ourselves short.

And so it is with our expectations of our own aging. It seems the only stories about aging successfully show ninety-year-olds running marathons or jumping out of airplanes. True, these people are most likely aging successfully, but just as you don't have to win a gold medal to be an excellent tennis player, we can age successfully without doing something that 99 percent of our peer group cannot. Likewise, aging well is much more than what the unenlightened stereotypes prevalent today say it is (e.g., we can expect more than to play bingo regularly).

So, if we can err by shooting too high or too low, how do we find the middle ground? Don't give up! Read on. I can help. Whether we act our age or not is determined by expectations, our own and others', so we need to discuss them.

The message of this chapter is simple: Don't let anyone else set the expectations for your aging. Just keep growing in all aspects of your life. No matter what the specific results are, you will be aging successfully.

Setting expectations is not all bad. We need goals or targets to shoot for. Goals provide us direction and a destination. They become problematic, however, when they become fixed and inflexible. If we set them too high, we will inevitably be disappointed. So, as in the case of the situations I mentioned in the opening of this section, we rob ourselves of the satisfaction of achieving some of our goals. Even more tragic than not achieving whatever expectation we had for ourselves is loss of the competence and pride that come with achieving something, anything. In most cases, I believe this sense of joy far outweighs the actual goal. If we are flexible, resetting expectations along our journey of growth, we can preserve this sense of accomplishment even as we fall short of our original goals.

A bar too low

We are a society obsessed with youth. We have a preference for portraying beautiful, youthful people in our ads, magazines, videos, TV shows, and movies, with the implication that it is only the young who are out there doing exciting things and living life. Even more disturbing than this unexamined obsession with youth is the stacking of the deck against older adults that occurs when we judge whether someone is old or impaired or "losing it" using criteria developed by young people. This youth-driven blindness virtually guarantees that growing old in our society becomes a dissatisfying, even dehumanizing, experience. Dr. Bill Thomas, an international expert on elderhood, observes that many within our society think of older adults as *broken versions of younger adults*. Ironically, this unenlightened view of aging results in markedly diminished expectations for the entire group of older adults. We lump all older people together as a group in decline as if the variability and diversity we see and expect in youth fades with age.

In Okinawa, if you ask an older adult how old she is, she will, in many cases, lie to you. An older Okinawan may very well tell you she is *older* than her true age. To be old in Okinawa is not only to be revered, but it is to be an essential part of the community and society: an envied source of wisdom and experience. This status comes with responsibilities, which remain as strong expectations for all Okinawans, no matter what their age. These expectations are rooted in the Okinawan concept of *yuimaru*, best translated as "reciprocity," and meaning that all are obligated to help others.[1] The older Okinawan is no less obligated than those younger. So although it may be that as they age they may need more assistance, it is also expected that they continue to assist others.

In our society, we have examples of remarkably vital, robust, and iconic older adults (usually celebrities), but they are clearly considered the exception. This is, in fact, why we see news stories of a parachuting George H. W. Bush and of marathon-running eighty-year-olds, because they are markedly inconsistent with our prevailing view of aging. And because we have low expectations, it is not surprising that over the last century we have observed a self-fulfilling picture of the aging process that is dominated by decline. Research on aging, and a new generation of older adults with expectations more consistent with this research, will rock our traditional views and significantly raise the bar. But it will take time.

So, with a still-prevailing view of aging as a decline-only process, we can easily set low expectations for ourselves. We can accept that it is unseemly or delusional to dress in younger clothes, to seek out new experiences, to continue to learn or try new things, to keep up with technology. Such behavior, we might easily believe, will demonstrate an unwillingness to gracefully accept our aging, will invite criticism that we are not acting in a way consistent with our station in life (or worse, that we are "losing it"), will set us up for disappointment, will show the world we are not *acting our age.*

Likewise, if we allow the diminished expectations of those close to us—family, friends, and peers—to determine our own expectations, we will undoubtedly set our bar too low and miss opportunities for continued growth. Even when given with the best intentions, the advice to "act our age" throws water on the embers of our potential. The fire of what still could be is extinguished and we ultimately settle into a world of privileges without obligations or purpose—a scenario now known to accelerate our own decline.

Where you live affects how you age—and how you expect to

As Masterpiece Living developed the tools to help older adults identify where they are at risk for not aging optimally and then to coach them toward better lifestyle choices, it became clear to us that this process was exponentially more successful when the individual was in a supportive environment: one that helped them believe in and *expect* continued growth. The *environment* was absolutely critical as a positive or negative influence on the outcome. People living where others were negative about aging or had only expectations of decline with aging, or in places where comfort and security were the dominant characteristics of the community, did not have the outcomes of those who lived in more nurturing environments. In communities where there was an overriding belief that older adults can continue to grow no matter what age or impairment, we saw startling growth: physically, intellectually, socially, and spiritually.

We knew that we now had to focus on helping to build these environments, and that focus paid off. Our Masterpiece Living network of nearly one hundred communities is a treasure house of what we hope will become models for communities of all types, including mixed-age, non-retirement communities. Creating places with village-like characteristics, no matter what the size of the community, is the goal. Creating places that respect and value older adults, that help them believe in their potential, and that incorporate them into the very fabric of the community is what Masterpiece Living has been doing, and is dedicated to continue. These are environments counter to the ageism-tainted ones still dominating our current culture, but they are precisely the environments where older adults flourish.

"Acting your age" in these places had to mean continuing to grow. This is, in fact, the reason many experts discourage living with one's adult children. On the surface it looks like a reasonable thing to do: Accept the love and protection of our grown children and let them assist us and free us of responsibility, right? It does indeed sound like a rational plan, but within these loving arms of our family, there are often entrenched and confining expectations of what you are capable of. There is a nurturing, albeit paternalistic, hovering that commonly characterizes this live-in arrangement. Appreciative of all you've done for them, expecting decline, and desiring to minimize, if not eliminate, the risk of injury, adult children and their families will often perform tasks that their parents are perfectly capable of doing. As we've seen in chapter 1, we lose what we do not use, and therefore, this time-honored, nurture-based approach to aging parents potentially raises risks.

And there's something else going on here. Years of playing roles as parent and child have left an indelible mark on both you and your children. There are expectations that come with those roles. Even as you age, your children expect you to be the solid, responsible, think-of-others-first person you were during your parenting years. Drift from this expectation, make efforts to grow or explore undeveloped areas of your personality, and you risk a family in chaos, and even suspicion that you are heading down the road to dementia! This can easily limit spontaneity and growth and therefore is potentially deadly to successful aging, even outweighing the social-connection benefit provided by the family.

Shake it up

So, whether we blindly adopt an unenlightened society's view of aging or the risk-averse view of those close to us, we short-change our growth and potential, and "act our age" all the way to decline and "usual" aging. In childhood we heard the admonition to act our age. In adulthood childish or adolescent behavior could have severe consequences, such as loss of job and relationships. But as an older adult, it's time to reconsider. The difference here is that acting our age for older adults is too restrictive and based on faulty assumptions. To age successfully in our current society, then, *requires* us to *never act our age*. It is not acting childish, but childlike. It is to do what Margaret Mead told us she did on her own aging journey: "I was wise enough to never grow up, while fooling most people into believing that I had."

It's not easy. As we age, we settle into comfort zones made very hospitable and inviting by our experiences. We've learned the "right" way of doing things, which quickly becomes the "only" way of doing things. We are more aware of the consequences of taking chances and easily adopt a conservative approach and attempt to eliminate all risk of failure, embarrassment, or criticism. We forget that to have a pulse is to be at some risk, that victory is sweeter when more is wagered.

Don't misunderstand. In Tip Five, I spoke about reducing your risk of disease and injury. And we should do that. But to avoid risk altogether is impossible and, when the most likely negative outcome is only embarrassment, avoiding risk is selling yourself short. Taking calculated risks, taking risk where the potential outcome is growth, joy, increased competence, and reduced risk of decline—that is an acceptable, even recommended, risk. In fact, I strongly recommend to my presentation audiences that they do something that scares them every day. It doesn't have to be bungee jumping or parachuting (although if that is where your heart is, go ahead—find a way to minimize the risk and go for it!). It must, however, take you out of your comfort zone. Remember, *we cannot grow if we don't change.* Change involves fear, especially if we take on too much. When you challenge your physical, mental, and emotional self, you grow. Your immune system, your brain, your muscles cannot help but respond to the challenge. You will be better and you will feel fulfilled. The challenge is clear: act your age and you risk suspension of growth. No growth equals decline as we age.

Turning the clock back

Dr. Ellen Langer, a Harvard University researcher, conducted a now famous study back in the late seventies. Using older men as subjects, she immersed them in an environment from twenty years earlier. Room trappings were from the fifties. Conversation about fifties-era topics was in present tense. Recorded radio programs were fifties vintage. This immersion resulted in the men acting in ways similar to their twenty-years-younger self: walking more, carrying their own luggage, doing things that had previously been done for them. The results after *only one week* were stunning: vision, hearing, cognitive skills all improved. Even photos of the subjects before and after the study improved, with subjects looking younger. What were Dr. Langer's conclusions? This work and a large body of research since this initial study convinces her that when we are aware—mindful of what we are doing and what expectations we have for ourselves—our bodies will follow; that is, *our bodies will attempt to align with those expectations.*[2]

To the extent we think of ourselves as more capable, or healthier, or growing, our bodies will attempt to reflect that view. Our bodies reflect our minds. The words of famous motivational speaker Brian Tracy—"You are what you think about"—reflect Dr. Langer's research conclusions. Her research has moved us way beyond euphemisms about being better if we try. We become better when we think of ourselves as younger, or more active, or more capable. Our brains begin to rewire to be consistent with a younger person. So, again, if we "act our age," within a context where being old is defined as declining, it's more likely that that is exactly what will happen. If, on the other hand, we act younger, more optimistic, more confident about what we are capable of, we will indeed grow and limit decline.

As I explained in the introduction to this book, Chuck Yeager taught me this many decades ago. Grandma Moses knew this when she began her painting career in her late seventies; Frank Shearer knew it when he celebrated his hundredth birthday by water skiing in Acapulco; Nola Ochs shouted it out to us as she received her undergraduate degree at ninety-five and master's degree at ninety-eight!

Perhaps F. Scott Fitzgerald was telling us much the same in his 1922 short story "The Curious Case of Benjamin Button," the basis for the 2008 movie of the same title, which starred Brad Pitt. Benjamin Button is born an old man and ages backward. Fitzgerald's powerful ability to articulate his sharp social insight provides us a story that holds our society's sclerotic views of aging up in sharp relief. Benjamin Button's experiences as a withered child and a robust older man challenges us to question our most entrenched concepts of aging.

Ethel shows us how

You remember Ethel. She is the theatrical dynamo we met earlier, who still writes a column for a New York publication targeted to older adults, and is involved with the Ms. Senior America pageant. When Ethel tells me "I never use a script," she is referring to her television talk show she hosted for many years in New York City. Hearing her story, however, I believe the words characterize something more significant. Ethel doesn't use a script for her life. Not society's script for an older woman, not her friends' script for their peer group, not anyone's. She follows her bliss, as Joseph Campbell told us to do. She does this spontaneously and fearlessly. How else could she have agreed to compete for Ms. Senior America at age sixty? Why else is she singing and directing a Broadway-type show at age ninety? How can she want to help others and to try new things after being widowed twice, surviving cancer, and being the caretaker for her husband? Yes, Ethel shows us how to age in a better way as she fully accepts her chronological age while raging against what she "should" be doing at ninety.

❧ Masterpiece Living Pearls for Never "Acting Your Age"

1. OK. Get back into your most comfortable chair. Think. *What would you do if you knew you couldn't fail?* It's an important question. The answer is something dear to you. Something that you no doubt have thought quite a lot about over the years, but most likely had let go when you became "too old." (I find it difficult to even type the words.) So what is it? Whatever it is, it's time to dust it off and consider doing it now.

   a) Maybe you wanted to swim the English Channel. Well, most of you wouldn't try it now, but how about doing it with a little adjustment? It's twenty-one miles from Dover to Calais, so why not set a timetable to accumulate twenty-one miles of swimming? Say, swim twenty-one miles in a month, or two weeks, or a week?

   b) Always wanted to run a marathon? Train for it and do it. Or walk 26.2 miles. Or set a timetable to walk the marathon distance.

   c) Always wanted to go to Antarctica? Well, go. Or take a course on it. Or listen to a lecture from someone who's gone. Or read more about it.

d) Always wanted to learn to play the guitar or piano or flute? Do it. You won't make Carnegie Hall, but do it anyway. Even if no one ever hears you. A new language? So many new ways to learn a language. No barriers but in your head.

2. What scares you? What have you avoided most of your life but would secretly like to have? Once you admit to what this is, decide that you will take my advice and scare yourself by beginning to take steps to decondition yourself. John Wayne said, "Courage is being scared to death but saddling up anyway." Afraid of public speaking? Try speaking while in front of a mirror. Try saying a few words the next time you are at a gathering of friends. Afraid to fly? Commit to a short flight. Speak to the person seated next to you and tell them you are afraid, and they will most likely talk you through the entire flight. Whatever it is that frightens and therefore limits your growth, you must identify it, realize that it presents an opportunity for substantial growth, and then begin taking baby steps to face your fear without having to fully face it until you're ready.

3. Consider traveling without making all arrangements and therefore leaving a few details to spontaneity. Looking back, some of the most memorable moments of my travels were unplanned. Yes, it might make you uncomfortable, but you will be proud when you pop through unscathed and more competent.

4. Just make a commitment to grow—to get a little better physically, mentally, socially, and spiritually. Just baby steps (see chapter 3). Then build on that. More baby steps. That alone breaks with the stereotype of aging as decline. Remember, age is a number—worth celebrating, then forgetting. It matters not so much where you end up, only that the journey is one of striving for growth.

WHEREVER YOU ARE . . . BE THERE

There are only two ways to live your life. One is as though nothing is a miracle; the other is as though everything is a miracle.

—ALBERT EINSTEIN

Nothing can give you joy. Joy is uncaused and arises from within as the joy of Being. . . . It is your natural state, not something that you need to work hard for or struggle to attain.

—ECKHART TOLLE

Life is so short we must move very slowly.

—THE TALMUD

When I was in my medical training, I was taught that if I could not bandage it, sew it up, treat it with medication, cut it out, or otherwise physically modify it, then it was not for me to attempt to heal. Only several decades later and after a career in preventive medicine did I learn what my medical school professors either didn't know or were reluctant to discuss. We cannot be truly healthy unless we are spiritually healthy. Yes, paying attention to our physical selves is a must, the foundation of our interaction with the world. Our intellectual component also needs our attention if we wish to experience our world fully. Social connection is key to reducing our risk of losing our independence. But spiritual health, I have come to believe, is the glue of it all, the road map of our journey, the thing that makes it all make sense. Viktor Frankl agreed: "The spiritual dimension cannot be ignored, for it is what makes us human."[1]

Dr. Harold Koenig, a physician at Duke University and an international authority on spirituality and health, tells us that spirituality is "the personal quest for understanding answers to ultimate questions about life, about meaning, and about relationship to the transcendent."[2] What is particularly appealing about Dr. Koenig's definition, unlike the hundreds of other attempts to define spirituality, *is that he believes it is a quest and not so much the destination.* Seeking answers to questions such as Why am I here? What is my relationship to other living things and to the transcendent? What is my purpose? What is the meaning of my existence?—this constitutes that quest. Seeking such answers is a spiritual journey, fundamental to who we are as humans, not something arbitrarily chosen by people with time on their hands. French philosopher Pierre Teilhard de Chardin grasped this concept: "We are not human beings having a spiritual experience. We are spiritual beings having a human experience." Perhaps, then, based on Koenig's definition, spiritual health is found in seeking answers to the fundamental questions of life. Or as Lewis Richmond said: "Spiritual practice is paying attention to things that matter." Certainly, as we age, we tend to be more contemplative and likewise more concerned with the spiritual. Thomas Moore, in his number-one *New York Times* bestseller *Care of the Soul: A Guide for Cultivating Depth and Sacredness in Everyday Life*, agrees: "Growing old is one of the ways the soul nudges itself into attention to the spiritual aspect of life. . . . The body's changes teach us about fate, time, nature, mortality, and character. Aging forces us to decide what is important in life."[3]

Lars Tornstam, a Swedish sociologist at Uppsala University, calls this period of advanced age *gerotranscendence* and describes it as "a shift in meta perspective, from a materialistic and rational view of the world to a more cosmic and transcendent one, normally accompanied by an increase in life satisfaction."[4]

In his inspiring book, *The Five Stages of the Soul*, Dr. Harry Moody is more specific about this spiritual journey of later life, describing it in five distinct stages, beginning with a realization that perhaps what seemed to be of value earlier in our lives is not, and progressing to a stage where we fully comprehend what does have lasting value for us and, as a result, find spiritual fulfillment.[5]

It's clear, then, that aging is associated with a metamorphosis for many of us, a call to search for meaning, value, peace, and if we're successful with this journey, joy.

So, what's stopping us?

Why is it, then, we may ask, that so many never find this joy, or even begin the journey? In the answer to this question lies a treasure trove of understanding, of wisdom, of mystical revelation and the meaning of life. This question is so fundamental that every religion, most philosophical theories, and many cults and political constructs have attempted to answer it. In the end, the answer is quite simple. The nearly universal obstacle to finding spiritual health is, ironically, ourselves.

The human brain is a magnificent organ that distinguishes us from all other living creatures. Our ability to reason, our memory, and our learning capability are all unparalleled, and as far as we know, not present in any other living creature. Some of these unique brain abilities, however, have doomed us to wander the earth, driven, confused, distracted, and detached. Why? Our minds are incessantly carrying on a conversation within us or in spite of us, much like an endless soliloquy from a Shakespearean tragedy. This chattering—or as our Buddhist friends call it, "monkey mind"—is a relentless battering of consciousness, which, because we all experience it, is considered normal. We, in fact, think we are our minds! Rather than considering our minds a tool of our magnificent human brain, we humans fully identify with the chattering and believe it is who we are. But we are so much more.

Our own worst enemies

We are souls, or spirits, or mystical creatures who have many exceptional capabilities, including a brain and mind that can reason, and judge, and talk longer than an adolescent girl on her cell phone. As the internationally known spiritual advisor Eckhart Tolle tells us, however, *we are not our minds.*[6] And as our mind rips around the racetrack of our consciousness, as it pulls us into an imagined or hoped-for future where we will have our to-do list completed, as it causes us to worry about all the possibilities for our own disaster or fantasize about being saved and finding our happiness, or as it yanks us back into the past with regret, or a preoccupation with what might have been—all these mental wanderings prevent us from being present in *this* moment, where life is lived, where the fulfillment we all seek is, where joy resides, where our journey begins and ends.

Perhaps even as you read this, your mind is leaping about the jungle of your consciousness. I'm getting tired. How long is this chapter? What makes him an expert? After this chapter I have to go to the store and pick up bread and milk. Didn't I read that somewhere else? My butt hurts. What's that noise? I should recommend this book to Andy. I could write a book if I wanted to. I feel like a beer. And on and on and on it goes, where it stops . . . We all experience this and therefore we don't see it as a sickness, or an affliction. We seek respite from this chattering—in sleep (unless we are one of the unfortunates who cannot shut off this chattering at night), alcohol, drugs, sex, or play. Many find peace in the rush of adrenaline and endorphins as they participate in dangerous activities such as racecar driving, mountain climbing, or bungee jumping. For when you are occupied completely with a life-or-death decision, your mind must be focused like a laser on what you are doing. And so it is ceases to chatter. And it is called "a rush," "exhilarating," and "thrilling," and yes, even "joyful." Because in those moments of awareness without thought lies what we all seek: spiritual fulfillment, peace, joy.

But of course, we needn't be pursuing death-defying activities to find the bliss Joseph Campbell urged us to find. Many find their fulfillment in faith, or nature, or music, or reading, or children, or the service of others. It is only when we can find the place Buddhists call "no mind," places where we are aware, even hyperaware, but without thought, that we experience the peace, fulfillment, and joy of being.

We have all found these places, however briefly. You witness a sunset, and the color and brilliance and silence completely captivate you, and all thought stops, and you feel that all is right in the world. Beautiful. And then it begins—the thoughts, the chattering, the monkey mind. Is this one as beautiful as the one I saw last September in Oregon? What would you call that color? That person with the camera is blocking my view. After this I have to eat. And the moment is gone. The peace and rightness of the moment is gone. And you are already moving on to your to-do list, or you're judging, or comparing, or worrying about whether the evening will go as you want it to. And you are no longer in the moment. You are being taken over by monkey mind.

Dr. Jill Bolte Taylor's *My Stroke of Insight*, as mentioned earlier, describes the author's experience with a stroke that essentially shut down the left side of her brain, which is the center of our incessantly chattering mind. While she was functioning with the right side of her brain, she experienced what she describes as pure joy, connection with all things in the world, a liberation, a euphoria she called "nirvana." As a neuroanatomist, she understands what happened to her, and in her many presentations since her recovery, she explains how each of us can actually choose where our consciousness spends its time. We can choose the right side of our brain and experience the joy of freedom from our incessant chattering minds, choosing to be "in the moment," if only for a short period.

My friends who are artists tell me they find "no mind" nearly every time they paint. Totally engrossed in what they are doing, totally aware of shadows, color, light, and lines, they become completely oblivious of time and feel a contentment, peace, or joy. This reaction is, in fact, reported by many in the creative arts, which enlist the right brain more than the left. When we are free of our sense of time and the frenetic activity that comes with it, we are rooted in *this moment* and our minds cease to race, and chatter, and rip us away from life as we feel it should be lived. Perhaps you have found it. Even if just for seconds, seeing your grandchild for the first time, taking time to notice a bird in your feeder, smelling a rose in the garden, meditating, or petting your dog. Many, of course, find these moments in prayer. These are the moments of spiritual fulfillment, of spiritual health. Finding them is critical, in fact, to aging successfully. If we cannot, we become victims to one of the most serious threats to a healthy aging experience: stress, the Big Uneasy.

Beware of the tiger within us: the Big Uneasy

As we evolved, our species developed a highly efficient mechanism for survival. Confronted with a threat, we fight or we flee. This fight-or-flight mechanism, the stress response, is associated with physiologic changes that enabled us to run faster or fight with more strength. We share this remarkable capability with our fellow mammals as well as lower forms. Faced with a threat to our survival, our levels of adrenaline and other neurotransmitters and hormones spike, with a resulting jump in heart rate, elevation of blood pressure, increase in breathing rate, surge of oxygen levels and blood glucose and fats, increase in blood-clotting ability, and shutting down of all nonessential systems in order to meet the challenge. All this is physiologically appropriate.

But in a world where immediate threats to life and limb are rare, shouldn't we be experiencing less stress? How is that so many of us admit to being "stressed out" and that the diseases of high stress, such as heart attacks, ulcers, and psychological disorders, are so prevalent? We wonder, as the title of Dr. Robert Sapolsky's compelling book asks, "Why don't zebras get ulcers?[7] His answer is clear. The stress response is meant to be fight or flight, mobilized in an emergency, and once the threat to the zebra is over (when he outruns the lion that was looking for dinner), the response dissipates. Shouldn't it be that way with us?

The answer would be a resounding yes except for our unique capability of generating a stress response with our thoughts. Yes, we as humans, with our more highly evolved brains, are capable of triggering this stress with *thoughts of danger or threat*. The zebra does not worry about the next lion threat. He is at ease after he has escaped. When we think of threats, or imagine ourselves as threatened, we can trigger mechanisms in the more primitive parts of our brain, those responsible for our fight-or-flight mechanism. Our chattering minds tell us we must finish our to-do list, or that the mole on our cheek might be melanoma, or that our grandson might be a drug dealer, or they take us into the future, where we might not have enough money for a long retirement, or where we might get cancer, or Alzheimer's disease. Or we go into the past and recall perceived grievances or missed opportunities or regrets. It's the equivalent of being constantly stuck in a cage with a hungry lion. The beast within—the Big Uneasy.

So what does our body do while we're getting more terrified or angry by the minute? You guessed it. We turn out the neurotransmitters and hormones that then whip our bodies into a frenzy so we can deal with a life-threatening situation. But wait a minute. There isn't a threat. We created one in our mind. So what happens when our bodies respond as if we're stepping on the gas and the brake at the same time? We beat ourselves up. We increase the possibility, especially if we are chronically under stress, of serious disease. Chronic stress places the cardiovascular system under considerable strain and compromises the immune system, decreasing our ability to fight off disease and other real-life threats. We say we are stressed, but more accurately, we are stressing ourselves. There is an analogy to help us understand the powerful negative effect of stress. The author of the analogy is unknown but the message is becoming familiar: Pick up a glass of water. It is light and easy to hold comfortably. Think of that glass of water as stress. Pick it up and put it down and there is little effect. Picking it up and holding it, however, for hours, days, weeks, or longer results in pain.

Our unique ability, or perhaps curse, to generate a stress response with our thoughts and reactions to a rushing, time-dominated world to which we have not yet biologically adapted is indeed one of the main themes of this book.

Beyond this physical stress, there's another dark side to our incessant mind talk. We tend to constantly judge, evaluate, and criticize anything that is not consistent with our deeply rooted beliefs. Any negativity, judgment, or criticism is a denial of what is, and therefore a source of stress, pain, and suffering. In fact, most spiritual teachings tell us that acceptance of the present—as it is, without judgment, resistance, or criticism—is true enlightenment. Spiritual teacher Eckhart Tolle writes, "All negativity is caused by . . . denial of the present. Unease, anxiety, tension, stress, worry—all forms of fear—are caused by too much future, and not enough presence. Guilt, regret, resentment, grievances, sadness, bitterness, and all forms of nonforgiveness are caused by too much past, and not enough presence."[8] Mark Twain recognized this over a hundred years earlier: "I am an old man and have known a great many troubles. But most of them never happened."

Seek out the now

And so we should seek presence; wherever we are, we can find it. Like the painter, we must seek a "place" where we can quiet our chattering, judging mind and experience *this moment*, this sacred moment, the only place our lives can be truly lived, free of the incessant mind noise that diverts us from finding spiritual health and fulfillment. Even if only for a moment, this liberation of our spirits breaks the spell of our uncontrolled thoughts and the pain, suffering, and stress they bring as their traveling mates.

To get there, we can paint, take a walk and be with nature, listen to Beethoven, spend time with a child, make furniture, or just sit and feel our bodies as we sit—the possibilities are many. Many find peace in practicing their faith. These people find spirituality in religion. Many others find spirituality in nonreligious places. It matters not. What does matter is that we find these places with quiet minds, places where we are completely in this magnificent moment life has given us. Whatever it is, this moment is what it is, and in this acceptance lie peace and joy. This doesn't mean we "roll over" and not attempt to deal with things, only that whatever we do, we begin with the total acceptance that this "thing" exists, and then fix it, leave it, or accept it.

Thomas Moore, in *Care of the Soul*, equates this search for quiet mind and presence to caring for the soul. "The soul," he says, "is not a thing, but a quality or a dimension of experiencing life and ourselves. It has to do with depth, value, relatedness, heart, and personal substance." He adds, "Soul cannot thrive in a fast-paced life because being affected, taking things in and chewing on them, requires time."[9]

Meditation is a powerful and ancient tool for orienting ourselves in this present moment. So simple yet with profound effects, meditation is the object of renewed interest, yet it still remains misunderstood by most of us in the West. Simply bringing our awareness to the present moment so completely as to nudge our ever-present thoughts into the background, meditation is a foreign concept to those of us who inhabit a frenetic, achievement-oriented world. Awareness without thought—simple and difficult.

Most meditation leaders advise sitting quietly and bringing awareness to the breath: not assessing how much or how fast, but just observing breathing in and out. Although to our get-things-done world this seems useless, frivolous, or even ridiculous, the result of spending time in a present, quiet place, even just seconds, will shock the most suspicious and skeptical of us. Brain research on meditation has documented its stimulus of the prefrontal cortex, which is associated with positive emotions, self-control, and even temperament.[10] Additionally, it is associated with "taming" the amygdala, which is the hub of fear memory, resulting in less likelihood of anger, frustration, shock, and even surprise.[11] Lastly, meditation is associated with a slowing of the shrinking of the gray matter of the brain normally associated with aging.[12] It appears, then, that quieting our chattering mind is not only associated with better health and aging but also, from an evolutionary standpoint, a more natural human state. In fact, as Eckhart Tolle tells us, we have never lived a moment that was not the present. We may have allowed our thoughts to remove us from that moment, but all life is lived in the present. The trick, then, is to spend more time there—i.e., to *be here*.

Mabes laughs

Mabes is ninety and has lived a life packed with more experience than five typical lives. She sums it up this way: "I was born laughing and I hope to die laughing." She grew up in an abusive household, the youngest of three. Her mother died under suspicious circumstances when Mabes was ten. When she was thirteen, she ran away from her home to live with her aunt and uncle. She also began working at thirteen in order to buy books for high school. Mabes graduated valedictorian of her class and won a scholarship to college. Just before she was to graduate from college, the Japanese attacked Pearl Harbor, and she decided to leave school to enlist in the military, but a professor convinced her she would be more valuable to her country if she had a diploma. Immediately after graduation, she joined the coast guard, went to officer training school, and became a search-and-rescue boat captain assigned to San Francisco Bay. She served until the end of the war and then joined the CIA. After an assignment in Italy, she was posted in Japan, where she met her husband and gave birth to her only child, her son. She accompanied her husband, who worked for the US State Department, to Spain, Argentina, Venezuela, and then back to the States, where after over twenty years of marriage, her husband filed for divorce.

Today, she lives in a retirement community in Delaware, and her son, her only family, lives in Seattle. Despite this, Mabes is not "retired" and refuses to be lonely. She drives a yellow VW Beetle, is currently learning Swahili, and is taking two other courses at the local college: "History of WWII" and "The Bible as Literature." She rides a stationary bike regularly, belongs to a book club, and crafts jewelry. She has traveled much, and not with tours. She has traveled by paddleboat in Ecuador, gone down the Amazon in a canoe, been to Italy to "restore" her Italian, and also traveled to Switzerland, Mexico, and parts of South America.

Recognizing that, as Mabes herself says, "we make our own heaven or hell on this earth," however, she has taken measures to preserve her inner peace. She watches no television (other than a sporting event six times a year), walks daily, and has decided not to use a computer. "I haven't sold my soul to any religion," she says, but she follows many of the beliefs of Buddhism. She is a vegetarian. But it is yoga, she says, that changed her life. Many years ago, she developed rheumatoid arthritis and began having difficulty moving. She discovered yoga in Venezuela and has actively practiced it for decades. She, in fact, teaches yoga to her neighbors three times weekly. In Venezuela, her teacher accepted no payment but the promise to teach yoga to others. She has done that, never accepting any payment for her instruction. She appeared on *The Today Show*, where she showed remarkably more flexibility than her two hosts, who were decades younger. Watching her teach, I saw her lean and flexible body do things I don't believe someone decades younger could do. Her face was serene and glowing.

When asked what advice she would give to others about aging, she quickly responds. "You can cope with anything. Things will get better if you help." She advises everyone to accept aging as part of life, but not to concentrate on it. "Keep playing, laughing, singing, dancing, and moving." To sum up, she smiles and says, "Make sure you *grow* old."

❦ Masterpiece Living Pearls for Being Wherever You Are

1. Learn to spot the threat. As Eckhart Tolle tells us, be the watcher of your mind. Rather than let your thoughts become the driver of your emotions and then of your physiology, observe your mind as it begins to get wound up with worry and negativity. Just observing your thoughts and mind puts you back in control so that those thoughts do not trigger the stress response, cause you to "lose it," or cause you to be removed from this important and sacred moment. Don't judge your mind, just observe. *Wow, look how my mind is getting itself all out of joint over this thing.* This reminds you that *you are not your mind* and therefore that you can guide and control what and how you think and, consequently, your stress response and whether or not you are *in the moment*, where the beauty and joy of life resides.

2. Look for those things that bring you comfort and joy. Not necessarily pleasure—that comes from outside of us—but joy, which comes from within. What activities cause you to lose track of time? To feel

totally in sync with the world? To feel contentment? To feel ener-gized? Is it painting, or a craft, or walking with the dog? Or perhaps listening to music, or reading, or observing nature, or being with your grandchild? Or is it being involved with your faith or doing another religious activity? Whenever you catch yourself feeling elated, free of the sense of urgency or time crunch, note it. And plan to spend time doing those things, even if you think they are silly or frivolous. Nothing is frivolous if it brings you closer to the mystery of a life fulfilled. Only you can discover and know what it is that will bring you this joy, and help you be wherever you are, rather than make you feel kidnapped by your chattering mind.

3. Consider meditation. As mentioned in Tip Three, meditation is associated with positive physical changes in the brain and may actually slow the brain atrophy that can come with age.[13] It's no big deal—really. All meditation requires is a few minutes to start with. You can sit on the floor on a cushion, but that's not necessary. You don't have to fold your legs up behind your neck. You can just sit up straight in a chair. Then, all you have to do is to focus your attention on your breath. "I'm breathing in. I'm breathing out." Very quickly your mind will start to do its thing: This is stupid. Am I doing this right? What's supposed to happen? When this occurs, and it will, guide your focus gently back to your breath and continue. Don't beat yourself up; just focus again, and again if necessary. Pay attention to your breath for two minutes and then extend the time as you get better. Or focus on a flower or a candle, and *see* it, study it, without judgment. Just notice the shadows, the color, the movement. You will find great peace and contentment as you are able to become more highly aware without thought, a time of "no mind," for longer and longer periods. You will feel less driven by your thoughts, and more in control. Pick up some instruction in meditation. You will find it both easy and rewarding.

4. Consider yoga, or tai chi, or qigong. Each of these has the power to calm your runaway thoughts, bring peace, and assist you to be present—i.e., to have awareness without thought. Additionally, they improve balance, strength, and flexibility—all important for aging successfully. Take a class, read some instruction, or have a friend show you. You will be delighted with the results.

5. As you go about your day, rather than have your chattering mind rush you to get things done, or worry, or think about anything other than what you are doing, take control. Be mindful, highly aware. As you climb stairs, feel your muscles as they lift you, be aware of breath being more rapid, pay attention to your arms. As you wash your hands, feel the water running over your fingers. Smell the soap. Be aware of your hand moving over the other hand. Your old self would have been absent from these actions, thinking of something else. Nothing would have been accomplished and you would have missed the great satisfaction and peace that comes with being there when you climbed the stairs, or washed your hands.

6. When you are attempting to be creative or solve a problem, every five minutes or so return to where you are. Be present, really see something around you, or feel your body sitting, or watch that tree limb move in the wind, and then get back to your problem solving or creating. You will find yourself more creative and the problem's solution will be more accessible.

7. When you encounter a problem, realize there are only three ways to deal with it: fix it if you can; walk away; or accept it. That's it. *Fix it, leave it, or accept it.* All else is madness and the source of pain, suffering, and stress-related disease.

8. *Give up the need to be right!* This trait, common to most of us, is alone responsible for prodigious amounts of pain and suffering, lowered quality of relationships, muted creativity, less effective work environments, and decreased overall quality of living. Begin today. On one small issue this very day, consider that you might be in error. Avoid building walls around your opinion and listen, *truly listen*, to the other possibilities and remain open to them.

9. Remember, you are not on this earth to rush around until you die. You are here to live your life, which can only be lived in *this moment*, not in the future or in the past or lost in racing thoughts.

FIND YOUR PURPOSE

Your happiness does not depend upon reaching your
goal, but upon setting a goal, and working toward it.
—JONATHAN LOCKWOOD HUIE

After I had made my presentation, the man approached me. He shook my hand with confidence and firmness. "You talk about purpose," he said. "Let me tell you, I worked damn hard my whole life. I was pretty successful, too." He waited for my nod before continuing. "Well, now I'm retired. My kids are all educated with good jobs and married. The dog just died, and . . . you know what?" My eyes inquired. "I don't need any more purpose. I'm done with that stuff."

My reaction to this was sadness. Where does this colossal misunderstanding come from? How can rational humans, having had purpose drive their entire lives, think that now they can wander through the rest of their lives with only comfort and recreation in mind? As if this post-retirement phase (which is getting longer all the time) is a cruise ship? Of course, it's easy to see why that might be appealing after decades of responsibility and struggle. After perhaps ten thousand days or more of rising from sleep with things to do, we can be easily seduced into thinking that living the rest of our lives without a to-do list would suit us. However, most of us cannot escape the need for a raison d'être.

Ultimately, our previous attachment to a purpose for getting out of bed in the morning will surface once again. Without a purpose, we are like a ship without a course, without a compass. We will run with the wind, and never feel the thrill of tacking into that same wind, making headway despite challenges.

Erik Erikson, in his classic 1950 book, *Childhood and Society*, defined eight stages of psychosocial development.[1] He explains that the seventh stage, Generativity vs. Stagnation, occurs between ages twenty-five and sixty-four and is characterized by many young-adult tasks, such as raising children and reversing roles with parents. However, there are several tasks that occur later in this time period: achieving mature social and civic responsibility, adjusting to the physical changes of aging, and using leisure time creatively. I believe that with the prolongation of life expectancy and the delay and redefining of retirement, these last tasks are now the work of people older than sixty-four. *Generativity* was defined by Erikson as "a concern for establishing and guiding the next generation," but he acknowledged that it could be expressed in many ways, including making a difference with one's life, or giving back, or taking care of one's community and planet. The main question of this period, then, is "Can I make my life count?" If indeed you accept that these are questions of older adults, then it is easy to see why a life of recreation, comfort, and security alone is likely to come up short when evaluated through the lens of generativity.

Indeed, in a later book, *Vital Involvement in Old Age*, Erikson identified this later-in-life generativity as "grand-generativity," a second opportunity "to incorporate care for the present with concern for the future, for today's younger generations and their futures, for generations not yet born, and for the survival of the world as a whole."[2]

The meaning of *meaningful*

Remember that one of the key characteristic of those who age successfully, according to the MacArthur Study was social connection, which was defined as having a network of friends and family, as well as continued meaningful activity. The word *meaningful* is key.

The Eden Alternative was founded by Dr. Bill Thomas to remake the environments for older adults needing care by recognizing the core belief that aging, even aging with impairments, should be a time of continued growth and development rather that decline. According to Dr. Thomas, "Meaningless activity corrodes the human spirit. The opportunity to do things that we find meaningful is essential to human health."[3] Key here is the phrase "things that *we find* meaningful."

Americans are an industrious lot. We work more hours than our European counterparts and hold productivity and outcome-oriented activity in very high regard. Add a salary to that and you've got the golden fleece of human effort. Which is why we often hear retired older adults explain that they "*only* volunteer" or "*only* work in my garden" or "*only* do some community theater." During their earlier years, these same people, like most Americans, obviously did not value such things as truly productive. Now, on the western side of their productive years, they are plagued by their own misunderstanding of what is meaningful. The value of any of our endeavors, and therefore their level of meaningfulness, can only truly be defined by each of us. You may choose to maintain earlier value systems of reimbursement or praise and may consequently experience the growing corrosion of your spirit. Or you may redefine value as something other than a capitulation or rationalization of your new status, realizing, based on the wisdom and experience you've gained during your life's journey, that enduring value might be different from your earlier assessment. Maybe what you value in life now includes a salary; maybe it doesn't. The key, again, is meaning.

Neuroscientists tell us that, unlike a younger person, who uses a focal area of the brain to solve a problem or make a judgment, an older adult uses much more of her brain for the same problem or judgment. This, they theorize, is the source of the wisdom of older adults. By incorporating more experience and brain faculties, the older adult sees a bigger picture. Rather than merely seeing the problem as an isolated challenge to meet and then move on from, the older adult sees it in the context of broader applicability. A driver pulls into the parking spot you've been waiting for. The younger person might lean on the horn, have harsh words, or move on to another space, angered by the ignorance and audacity of the other driver. An older adult might consider the possibility that the other driver didn't see her, or is much more harried, or has less social responsibility, or is potentially violent, or just that it's not that important to "win." A broader context.

So, too, a broader context should define our sense of what is meaningful. We should not be prisoners of previous, often unexamined, value systems. If an activity is meaningful to you, it will provide you with the continued engagement in life necessary to age successfully. This is another meaning of being authentic. To achieve authentic health we must be true to who we are, not only as a species, but also as individuals. Whether it's growing roses or lobbying to eliminate land mines, feeding birds or being politically active, picking up litter or saving the whales, you are the judge, the ultimate authority on what has meaning for you and therefore what will bring you satisfaction and even joy, and with that, a better aging experience.

Giving back

There is a scene in the movie *The Bucket List* where Morgan Freeman relates to Jack Nicholson that in ancient Egypt, in order to enter heaven, each person was asked two questions: Have you found joy in your life? Has your life brought joy to others? In conversations with hundreds of older adults, I have found that what brings meaning and purpose to lives—consistently, if not unanimously—involves other living things. Whether other humans, animals, plants, or the environment as a whole, living things give us a sense of giving back, of improving the lives of others or the planet, that particularly resonates with older adults. This is, of course, compatible with Erikson's view of grand-generativity. Dr. Albert Schweitzer told us, "I don't know what your destiny will be, but one thing I know: the only ones among you who will be really happy are those who have sought and found how to serve."

A comprehensive 2007 review of the research on the health benefits of volunteering found lower mortality rates, greater functional ability, and lower rates of depression later in life in those who volunteered, even those who did as little as two hours a week, compared to those who did not volunteer. Older volunteers were most likely to receive greater benefits because "volunteering provides them with physical and social activity and a sense of purpose at a time when their social roles are changing."[4] Our Masterpiece Living data also shows that volunteerism improves memory and the ability to provide help and support to peers. We were very pleased to see volunteerism rates consistently twice as high in our successful aging communities compared to national norms.[5]

A more recent study from the Universities of North Carolina and California–Los Angeles demonstrated that subjects whose happiness was based on a sense of higher purpose and service to others had gene expression profiles that were associated with augmented levels of antibody production and lower levels of pro-inflammatory markers (linked to cancer, diabetes, and cardiovascular disease). Those whose happiness came from consuming things had more unhealthy profiles.[6]

Mary Donnelly is eighty-three but is a phenomenon on Block Island, a small island thirteen miles off the coast of Rhode Island. A nurse for over fifty-three years on the island and the mother of seven, she has led a life filled with meaning and purpose. Now, in her ninth decade, she continues her volunteer work as the sole administrator of the Mary D. Fund, which aids full-time residents of Block Island when financial difficulties knock. She is a woman with a mission to help others.

Some enlightened senior living organizations have recognized the positive effects of volunteerism and have incorporated humanitarian efforts into the culture of the community. American Baptist Homes of the West (ABHOW) has a robust Social Accountability program that promotes outreach into the surrounding community. One senior-living community developed a garden with the help of 120 volunteers and then donated the produce they grew to a local food bank.

Purpose is not stagnant. As Richard Leider tells us in his book *The Power of Purpose*, "purpose is not discovered once and then we are done with it. It is reexamined at various points throughout the life cycle, typically during crises and major live transitions."[7] Precisely, and is not older age—a time when our current society tends to "pasturize" its older adults, putting them "out to pasture" with no expectations other than to enjoy retirement—a time of crisis for people who have succeeded in careers, raised children, owned businesses and homes, been mentors, helped raise grandchildren, and now are marginalized by that same society they helped build? Yes, this is indeed a time of potential major crisis. Ultimately, as our understanding of aging and what it takes to age successfully become more widespread—and as the content of this book and similar research, like the Masterpiece Living data on thousands of older adults, become common knowledge for policymakers and aging individuals—our society will begin to tap into the enormous resource that resides in our older adults. Until then, it will be up to each one of us to find what brings us meaning and purpose and to ascribe our own value to whatever it is we feel we must do to not only get out of bed in the morning but to move out from the pasture and onto life's pathways. And as we search for that path of meaning and purpose, we would do well to heed the advice of Mark Gerzon in *Coming into Our Own*: "If it feels safe, it's probably not the right path, but if it scares you, it probably is."[8]

Ray hums

Ray just turned eighty. He is African-American, is one of thirteen children in his family, served twenty years in the Air Force, and has a life-long interest in painting. Despite the fact that he has seen the worst of racial prejudice in his lifetime, he has consistently remained positive in his outlook on life. Having weathered the death of June, his wife of fifty-five years, as well as the onset of neuropathy in his legs, which necessitated that he use a walker, and having recently finished treatment for throat cancer, he attributes his resilience to focusing on the positive: "I could mope and groan and feel sorry for myself, but I still have things to do."

Ray's reputation and now contribution to the community is his success in leaving his walker in the fitness room. With a determined effort to walk better, he began a long commitment to get stronger and more flexible, which resulted in his walking today unassisted and with little evidence of the neuropathy that persists. Having seen the virtual miracle of his own effort, his purpose in life, his *thing*, is "to help as many people as I possibly can." As a passionate champion of exercise as a way to maintain independence, he encourages his neighbors to move more, even leading the morning exercise classes in his community when the regular instructor is not available. An older neighbor recently abandoned her wheelchair after working with Ray and the community's fitness expert.

When asked what he would tell younger people about aging, Ray advises them to "learn as much as you can about everything you can so that you can be in a position to assist someone else. I learned this from my mother and father. Do things with a good heart." That is Ray's clearly stated purpose and it shines through brightly as a guiding light in his young, aging eyes. His closing words to me in our conversation resonated: "I love to sing. Since my throat cancer surgery, I can't sing anymore, so I hum."

❧ Masterpiece Living Pearls for Finding Your Purpose

Your purpose lies within you. Dig deep and live your legend.

1. Imagine you're at your own funeral. A close friend or a family member is giving your eulogy. What would you like to hear? What would make you feel proud of your life? Of your accomplishments? What one thing would you particularly like to hear above all others? This one thing is something you should consider focusing on now. What can you do now to make sure that it's part of your life's legacy?

2. Ask yourself, "What is the work I cannot *not* do?" What is it that's been with you, weighed down by the "stuff" of your everyday life, but that every now and then floats to the surface, making you think *What if?* or *Wouldn't that be great?* Sever the weight that keeps it submerged and let it come to the surface. Begin to think *Why not?*

3. Don't discount that what you've been doing, whether it's paid work or volunteer work, may be bringing significant meaning and purpose to your life. However, be aware of the warning of Socrates: "The unexamined life is not worth living." Laziness and fear are strong motivators to keep on truckin' even when what you're doing is not "making your life count."

4. If you had $10,000 to give away to a cause or organization, which one would it be? Perhaps it's time to start or continue working for that cause or organization or something related to it. This is something meaningful to you and it obviously beckons you.

5. What did you want to do with your life when you were in your teens or early twenties, before life's responsibilities took root and determined your path? Consider researching this area and finding opportunities to work or volunteer in it. These youthful dreams often still hold a fascination, and returning to them can be very fulfilling.

6. If nothing resonates with you after going through these first five exercises, consider an exploratory period or trying new things that sound appealing. Pick up a new or long-neglected hobby. Consider volunteering. Take a class. Take a retreat from your daily life, preferably in a quiet natural setting (Native Americans called these "vision quests"). While there, allow your thoughts to wander freely, and see where they lead you.

7. Give up the idea that a purpose must be grandiose. You should not have to brag about your purpose or expect others to consider you saintly or heroic for pursuing it. The only real characteristic of true purpose is that it has meaning *for you* and brings you contentment and joy. No one else can tell you what is meaningful to you. You are the ultimate authority on what your purpose is. Yes, seeking a new purpose can be scary. It involves change. It *should be scary*, but if you are true to yourself as you seek it, you will find not only that purpose but also your authentic self, your life's definition, and a sense of satisfaction that will sustain you through the rest of your life's journey.

8. If you are adventurous, the Peace Corps—or the Peace Corps alternative, Cross-Cultural Solutions—and AmeriCorps have no upper age limits! Doing something that scares you will most certainly give you a sense of purpose.

HAVE CHILDREN IN YOUR LIFE

The soul is healed by being with children.
—FYODOR DOSTOYEVSKY

Walt Disney Studios has given us two markedly different views of the relationship between children and older adults in two award-winning animated movies: 1942's *Bambi* and the 1994 block-buster *The Lion King.* In the well-known story of Bambi, a young deer attempts to survive in the forest after the death of his mother with the help of some wise and playful young friends and a distant, yet all-pow-erful stag called the Great Prince of the Forest. The Great Prince remains aloof, swooping in when he's needed most, to tell Bambi he won't be able to be with his mother anymore and to save him from a pack of wolves, but then disappearing to live his own life, leaving Bambi to his own devices. It is apparent that the Great Prince believes the young deer will learn the lessons of life in the school of hard knocks. Bambi has adven-tures, learns how to survive, and eventually grows to adulthood.

I first saw *Bambi* as a very young child of five and was confused by the unwillingness of the Great Prince to teach Bambi all that he needed to know. The stag could have told him where to find water, good food, and safe places to rest or how to avoid predators. Why didn't he stay with Bambi and make his world so much safer? I also wanted to know more about the older buck. How did he get to be the Great Prince?

What battles had he had? How had he survived? What happened to his parents? But my questions were left unanswered and I felt fearful throughout most of the movie. (In the 2006 sequel, *Bambi II*, the relationship is less mysterious. The Great Prince tells Bambi that he will grow stronger and more resilient alone; ultimately, he becomes a loving parent to Bambi. Perhaps the angst of generations of young children finally made its way to the screenwriter.)

Now, as a grandfather, I look back on *Bambi* and have a changed point of view. Seeing the movie through the eyes of the older deer rather than Bambi's, I recognize the loneliness and isolation of the Great Prince. I know that if he could overcome whatever stiff and sterile notions he had of the relationship between older adults and children, there would be a treasure trove of wonder, optimism, joie de vivre, and forgotten values waiting for him. There would be the opportunity to play again, to shed the imposed and self-inflicted burdens of adulthood, and to be once more in *this* moment, with *this* child, sharing *this* gift of life, with nothing else to complicate that simple truth. With nothing else to cause him to pass adult judgment on the moment; to pull his thoughts away; to cause him to succumb to the siren voices of responsibility calling him toward the rocky shore of life without children, calling him to his own emotional death. I feel empathy and pity for the Great Prince of 1942, and celebrate his triumph in the enlightened 2006 sequel.

In *The Lion King* we have some similarities: Simba is a young lion making his way in the world under the watchful eye of an adult Lion King and some wise and playful friends. The Lion King has responsibilities and maintains a regal posture, even swooping in to save the young lion when he makes a bad judgment resulting in mortal danger, but the relationship is much more than that. The Lion King is engaged with the young cub, teaching him, scolding him, but also laughing, joking, and playing with him. The Lion King clearly is enriched by the interaction when he seizes the opportunity to drop his kingly demeanor, if only for a short time.

There is, in addition to this captivating story, a message of profound significance here: *the circle of life*. A clearly stated belief in the ongoing influence and stabilizing effect of intergenerational relationships; a philosophy that we are part of a dynamic, yet constantly repeated progression through life's stages; that we are related—in fact, inextricably so—to the generations that have preceded us and that will follow us; and that we are defined by this relationship.

A circle of connection and health

Most of us readily accept our responsibility for caring for our children and grandchildren. Today, with the disappearance of the village society (even the disappearance of the neighborhood of my own youth), there is a diminished responsibility for others' children. Of course, most people treat other people's children kindly but harbor a reluctance to offer more than a smile and greeting. If another person's child comes in direct opposition to the perceived happiness or health of our own, a fierce protectionism arises. The seemingly rising rate of child predators and an increasing rate of helicopter parenting (parents hovering over children as they move through life—an approach the Great Prince as well as the Lion King would surely take exception to) make interaction with children other than those in our own family less fluid and, in fact, less likely to happen at all. We have, therefore, scores of older adults who have no access to children because they have no children in their family. Scores of older adults disconnected from the circle of life and enriching, health-promoting relationship with the young.

Once again, it should not be surprising that we humans might be drawn to children. For eons, we gathered together in small, generationally diverse groups in order to survive in harsh environments. The flourishing of children not only ensured the survival of us as a species, or as a village, but also provided workers, soldiers, craftsmen, mothers, cooks, scholars, and all sorts of other human resources. Children were not only recipients of parental and village nurturing and instruction but also had crucial roles in the operation of the family and the society. We look back now and cringe at child labor and other unscrupulous practices that resulted from this accepted view making its way into the Industrial Revolution. In any case, children were an integral part of the human effort to survive and of the operation of the tribe; therefore, a life devoid of children is an anomaly.

But are children necessary to age successfully? Dr. Bill Thomas, founder of the Eden Alternative, once again weighs in. He firmly believes that elders must live in habitats for human beings, not in sterile institutions. The Eden team is dedicated to eliminating the plagues of loneliness, helplessness, and boredom that make life intolerable, believing that close and continuous contact with plants, animals, and children provides relationships that offer a pathway to a life worth living. According to Dr. Thomas, Eden Alternative homes report benefits to this approach, including reduction in medication use, lower mortality rates, less staff turnover, and fewer employee accidents.

Health insurer Humana sees the value of association with children. In association with KaBOOM!, a nonprofit that aims to build a playground within walking distance of every child's home, Humana has sponsored multigenerational playgrounds with equipment suitable for all ages. These playgrounds combine the benefits of physical activity and mingling with children in order to maximize the benefits of exercise and to help motivate older adults to move. These spaces will soon be in ten major cities.[1]

And what about the children? Do they benefit from the association with older adults? Big Brothers Big Sisters of America reports that children in their programs, after only eighteen months, were . . .

- 46 percent less likely to begin using illegal drugs
- 27 percent less likely to begin using alcohol
- 52 percent less likely to skip school
- 37 percent less likely to skip a class
- 33 percent less likely to hit someone[2]

Clearly this young people–older people association can be characterized as "win-win."

Brazil has launched an initiative to promote an active and healthier aging process nationwide. One strategy involves the development and promotion of multigenerational programs. One study involved students twelve to eighteen years old meeting with thirty-two elders for two-hour sessions once weekly for fourteen weeks. The joint activities involved memory sessions (storytelling and question-and-answer sessions), celebrations (birthdays), and the production of books and posters. The participating older adults showed positive quantitative changes in family relationships and the perception of social support. Positive effects were seen in the youth also.[3]

The value of intergenerational exchange is becoming mainstream in the healthcare community. The Intergenerational Center of Temple University's College of Health Professions and Social Work in Philadelphia recently won the Eisner Foundation's first Eisner Prize for Intergenerational Excellence for its Project SHINE (Students Helping in the Naturalization of Elders). The goal of Project SHINE, according to the

Intergenerational Center's founder and executive director, Nancy Henkin, is to "bring together young and old so everyone can feel like they're contributing to society from birth until death." Project SHINE brings together local immigrants who are struggling with integrating into the community and students through educational programs, volunteerism, and mentoring. This program has been a great success and has expanded to thirty-one colleges and two hundred ethnic community organizations. As Henkin says, "We're all in this together and our destinies are linked.[4]

Children as spiritual advisors

As I was about to become a grandfather over a decade ago, I had an idea that this would be a wonderful experience. Seeing my daughter as mother, a new child born into the world, a child I could enjoy but not have to raise myself—all great, right? Wrong! Not because it wasn't all those things, but because it was so much *more* than those things. It was, in fact, a mystical experience.

First, I had a profound sense of being part of an ancient, reoccurring, and soulful human drama. Actually, even beyond human in the sense that it is life being lived, life realizing its highest potential. The birth of Jackson sent me off on a metaphysical merry-go-round, which resulted in a gut understanding of the circle of life and my place in it. No abstract concept of birth, life, and death here, but the raw, naked understanding that comes to an existential player who is willing to take on many roles. Shakespeare's words from *As You Like It* seem apt:

> All the world's a stage,
> And all the men and women merely players:
> They have their exits and their entrances;
> And one man in his time plays many parts.

Even Shakespeare's words come up short. Suffice it to say, becoming a grandfather was a spiritual experience. Even more surprises came later. As Jackson began to notice, then recognize, then communicate, then play, and then befriend me—this was a validation that made the rewards of career and accomplishment pale in comparison, a validation of my very existence, of my role in this magnificent journey of life.

We can experience the Family of Man, or even the participation in a Life Force, with our relationship with other adults. With children, however, whether they arise from your own DNA or whether they merely share the core genome of all humans, our sense of place and role is sharpened, unveiled, as with a masterpiece on canvas hidden under a more mundane painting. Children are indeed the bearers and promoters of our more noble human qualities.

On a more practical level, children reduce our stress. Of course, many parents wouldn't agree, but that is precisely the point. When we can look beyond the complex parent-child relationship, with its focus on safety, discipline, and providing for needs, we can allow the relationship to be what it is, if only for short periods of time: two humans, in different places on a circle, yet connected, and both necessary to maintain the circle of life. We can then allow for a mix of unbridled optimism and experiential skepticism, of boundless energy and growing fatigue, of curiosity and experience, of innocence and wisdom. The result of this recipe is not always predictable, but it is healthy and satisfying and stress reducing, because when we are with children and not burdened of the duties and responsibilities of parenting, we are *with them*. We are less likely to be anywhere else. Not worrying about the world, or our aches and pains, or our finances, or our life expectancy. We are more likely to be in the moment with them and free of our self-induced stressors.

There is a widespread tendency to believe that modern children don't want to be with older adults. This is the logical conclusion of a smoldering ageism in our society. As noted above, the relationship between the old and the young is primal. It is the result of eons of tribal and village connection, which is encoded into our very DNA. Yes, it may require that we dust off, or even scrub off, some of the trappings of our modern era, but underneath, like the hidden masterpiece, is the prize.

Martin's mission

Martin is nearly ninety, a widower, and a retired aircraft company executive. He lives in a retirement community in Florida. He's gregarious, and optimistic. He plays tennis regularly and attends the local university's lifelong-learning classes. As a single man in a community where women outnumber men by as much as three to one, and where a major criterion for appeal is being able to drive at night, he's a rock star. But despite all this he was feeling empty. His grandchildren were grown, and he felt all he was doing was merely recreational, without purpose or meaning.

Martin was in charge of training for his company when he was still working and had always harbored a dream of being a teacher. So, one day, on a whim, he walked over to the local elementary school and went to the guidance counselor's office. He asked if there were any children who were struggling and whom he might be able to tutor. Luckily, the counselor was not closed-minded and paired him up with a struggling fifth grader, Brian. They began meeting once weekly at school and soon were meeting after school to enjoy a hot dog or go to a movie. Brian's grades began to improve, and the counselor approached Martin about possibly seeing other students and asked whether there were more older adults who might be interested in helping students. And so was born the mentor program.

Once weekly, Martin and forty of his neighbors set up forty card tables in the dining room of their retirement community and wait for the school bus to arrive with forty students. They pair off and spend the next hour talking—about school, math, history, and life. The school reports that the students are doing better in their studies and that there is a marked reduction in behavioral problems. Meanwhile, Martin and his neighbors spend a good part of the week preparing for the meeting. They are planning a big party for the last day of school, and many are going to meet with their young friends over the summer. Martin is happy. He has a bounce in his step, and has secretly started a bank account in Brian's name, which he hopes will be used as tuition for college. He knows, of course, that he won't be alive to see Brian in college, but he's proud nonetheless of Brian and cherishes their friendship.

ᴥ Masterpiece Living Pearls for Having Children in Your Life

1. Are you ready for younger people in your life? A little uncertain about whether you're ready or whether there are any kids out there who'd be interested in spending any time with you? Start slow. Spend time with children in your family if possible. Listen, observe, smile. Be relaxed. Show no signs of impatience or of having another place to go. The greatest gift we can give children is our time.

2. If you have no children in your family, try going to a children's movie (you might consider going with a friend given today's high

sensitivity) or a playground or any place where children are, in order to observe and get sampling of their energy. Still interested?

3. Contact the local Big Brothers Big Sisters and inquire into the requirements to enter their program. These organizations usually pair younger adults with children but are not limited to that model.

4. Visit the local elementary school and see if it's possible to become a mentor, or storyteller, or aide. Many schools' history classes will welcome an eyewitness account of twentieth-century events you have lived through. Such an offering frequently leads to other possibilities at the school, such as teacher's aide, or class grandfather or grandmother.

5. Inquire at the local library for any need for a children's storyteller or reader. Most libraries have active programs for children and will welcome your participation.

6. Go to the local hospital's children's ward to see if they have need for volunteers. Many welcome baby rockers. My mother knitted caps for newborn infants. By the time she had to give up knitting due to arthritis, she had provided caps for hundreds of newborns.

7. Do you have a special skill that could benefit children? Woodworking? Knitting? A musical instrument? Language? Local organizations such as Boys & Girls Clubs, community centers, the YMCA, the YWCA, church groups, summer camps, and other community-based organizations are hungry for volunteers and instructors.

8. Of course, the Internet is a valuable source for volunteering with children. My mother, Marguerite, made over a hundred small teddy bears for children in war and in storm-ravaged countries. She never saw these children but felt enriched even by this anonymous association. Other possibilities are pen pals and financial sponsorship for children in third-world countries.

LAUGH TO A BETTER LIFE

Laughter is the shortest distance between two people.
—VICTOR BORGE

Norman Cousins reacted the way any of us would have on hearing he had an incurable, crippling illness. There was the shock, denial, and anger. But then, he broke from the rest of us. He decided he could not be a passive observer of his own health. Norman Cousins began to laugh.

Why not? he thought. He was feeling pretty low and wanted to feel better. He knew laughter always made him feel physically, emotionally, and psychologically better, so why not laugh now? He had read in Hans Selye's classic 1956 book, *The Stress of Life*, of how stress and negative emotions could cause negative chemical changes in the body.[1] Couldn't positive emotions, then, cause *positive* chemical changes? Why not laugh and see if this was possible?

Of course, most of us could think of a lot of reasons why not, but Norman, a journalist, editor, and world-peace activist, looked at his situation differently. In his 1979 book, *Anatomy of an Illness*, he describes how after his diagnosis of ankylosing spondylitis, a degenerative disease of the spine, he rented a movie projector, Marx Brothers movies, and old episodes of *Candid Camera*.[2] He recognized almost immediately, after just ten minutes of laughing, that his pain was better. He continued to laugh. He laughed, and laughed, and laughed himself into remission for nearly thirty years, finally succumbing to heart disease. His physicians had no explanation for his remission. Could laughing have been responsible?

Laughing at 100

Results from the Boston University–based New England Centenarian Study indicate that it's possible to laugh yourself to better health, aging, and even longevity.[3] A preliminary conclusion of this fifteen-year-plus study is that those who live to be a hundred or more seem to be able to handle stress better than the majority of people. These are people who have lived long enough to experience significant loss in their lives, so they are realists. Yet, they believe they will meet whatever lies ahead when the time comes, so there's no need to fret about it now. (This is consistent with the "living in the present moment" approach we discussed in Tip Seven.)

Laughter researcher Robert Provine tells us that laughter is a primitive attribute, "an unconscious vocalization," and he considers it a "universal human vocabulary."[4] It is observable to some degree in other primates and is present in babies even before they can speak. Babies laugh as much as three hundred times per day, as opposed to us more somber adults, who average twenty times per day. Laughter is considered by most to be a human behavior and is strongly associated with positive human connection and social interaction, being part of a group. We have discussed social connection as a lifestyle characteristic strongly associated with successful aging, and so it would seem very consistent to associate better health with laughter. So what could be going on here? Can laughter somehow change our physiology?

Laugh power

Drs. Stanley Tan and Lee Berk of Loma Linda University have been studying the effects of "mirthful laughter" for over three decades. They have consistently demonstrated that laughter reduces stress hormones, which are known to suppress immunity. Conversely, laughter activates T cells, immunoglobulins, and natural killer cells, which collectively play a role in rejecting tumors and cells infected with viruses, as well as protecting us from infection. Laughter also increases beta-endorphins, which improve mood, reduce pain, and increase relaxation.[5] The bottom line? Laughter seems to boost our immune system, which has the potential to assist us in resisting cancer and infection, as well as a number of other threats to our good health and successful aging, and we feel much better while all this is happening.

Beyond immunity, laughter is therapeutic for those who are experiencing pain. A recent research report from Oxford demonstrated elevated pain thresholds after episodes of "laughter till it hurts" in groups. The mechanism, Dr. Robin Dunbar, the lead investigator, concluded, is the release of endorphins, the morphine-like substances produced by our brains in the pituitary gland and hypothalamus, and which give us pain relief and a general feeling of well-being. Dr. Dunbar, an evolutionary psychologist and anthropologist, also concluded that social laughter plays a key role in social bonding.[6] So, once again, we are reminded of the authentic needs we developed in our infancy as a species.

In addition to these positive effects, laughter is an "internal workout," contracting the diaphragm and abdominal muscles and providing us some relaxation. We all recognize that it provides a physical and emotional release. Lastly, as noted above, it is a social connector, improving the quality of social interaction while enhancing the mood of those sharing the laughter.

Dr. Berk states that "the best clinicians understand that there is an intrinsic physiological intervention brought about by positive emotions such as mirthful laughter, optimism and hope. Lifestyle choices have a significant impact on health and disease and these are choices which we and the patient exercise control relative to prevention and treatment."[7]

Choosing or losing

The Dalai Lama, in his book *My Spiritual Journey*, calls himself a professional laugher.[8] Despite the many difficulties he has faced as a Tibetan leader in exile, he chooses to look at life "holistically"—i.e., from many perspectives—to focus on the always-present positive aspects, and to laugh easily.

Ellen Langer, the previously mentioned prolific researcher and author and professor of psychology at Harvard University, has spent her career demonstrating that by being attentive and mindful and aware, we can be healthier. She believes that the placebo effect is real. When we physicians prescribe "sugar pills," a treatment without documented effectiveness, and the patient gets better, we conclude that the illness was not real; the symptoms were imagined. In fact, the placebo effect is a powerful tool in the physician's medical bag to help people feel better. Sir William Osler was a Canadian physician of the late nineteenth and early twentieth century and one of the founders of the Johns Hopkins University School of Medicine, and often called the "Father of Modern Medicine." He, too, believed in the power of the placebo, acknowledging that patients become well because of their faith in the effectiveness of treatment.

Dr. Langer believes that to the extent we believe and focus on getting better, we actually change our brains and then our physiology and program our return to health.[9] This same belief is the core of much of the positive psychology movement, which in turn drives a large segment of the motivational and self-improvement industry. Self-improvement icons Brian Tracy and Jack Canfield tell us that we are what we think about.

So, to the extent that we laugh, readily and often, we are doing much more than presenting a positive image to the world. We are, it seems, programming ourselves to be happy and healthier, and we're having fun doing it! There are many who believe that life is a head game. We choose to be happy; we choose to be positive. Likewise, we can choose to be unhappy and negative. Yes, life will throw us curveballs, challenges, and losses. It is an absolute certainty for those of us who have a pulse. As humans, unlike our brother and sister mammals with less developed cerebral cortexes, how we respond to these losses, what our minds choose to focus on, can make all the difference. We can beat our breasts and be a "woe is me" victim, or we can be like Norman Cousins and laugh. Laughing draws others to us. It increases our social connectivity, which, as we noted in Tip Four, is associated with higher likelihood of health and better aging. And, let's face it: in the end, it's more fun.

George on laughter

George is ninety-eight and living in assisted living at a retirement community in Palm Beach Gardens, Florida. He is a CPA and has never studied the research on aging or laughter. He uses a walker to help him maneuver about his apartment. His wife, Helen—"She was a doll, I tell you"—is gone. His brothers are gone. He has no children. This would seem to be that sour spot of life we all fear. Alone, impaired, and in George's own words, "on death row."

George's response to all this? "So what? You know you're going to die. You knew that when you were born. Why worry about it? I look at life the way I looked at my financial statements. I project for the next year. I look ahead."

In the two hours we spent together, George's laughter flowed freely. Even as he spoke of Helen's illness as a young woman, which drove them to be legally declared paupers; of her dementia in later life, which had her saying to him, "I never married you"; of the night she was wandering and fell, and he fell, and neither of them could get up because they both had fractures—interspersed between his recounting of all these "low points" in his life, George laughs. When he openly tells me he knows his father didn't want him because they couldn't afford the six kids they already had, he immediately adds, "but I came into the world for free" (the doctor never charged for his birth) and laughs. The staff tells me how George posted flyers reading "Smile" in several locations about the community. He teaches courses for his neighbors in assisted living, with materials he gathers from the Internet: a course on the earth from the big bang to five hundred years from now ("always looking ahead") and travel information about the countries of Europe. "I've done Visions of Italy," he says. "I'm going to get Visions of France and Greece and teach those soon."

George's laugh is infectious and accompanied by sparkling eyes and a broad smile. Despite his limited mobility today, he speaks with youthful energy and shares details about a two-month-long driving and camping trip he and his wife took over seven decades ago; how they enjoyed taking the Polar Bear Express in Canada; how Helen chased away a panther who was attempting to eat their dinner when camping. In a tour of his apartment, he proudly tells me of how he became an official Kentucky colonel. He shows me a building he designed, and, showing me wedding rings mounted in a frame, he adds, "She's still with me." And when I ask him what he would like to tell a younger person, he smiles. "Don't think about aging. It doesn't mean anything. You're living. That's what counts. You're living. You're enjoying life. I can run a program and it challenges my brain. I can work on it and have a lot of fun. I am a happy man. How?

Be busy, have a goal and work on it." And, of course, he closes this advice with a deep belly laugh.

❧ Masterpiece Living Pearls for Laughing to a Better Life

1. Look in the mirror. That's right. Look at yourself. You'll immediately want to suck in your gut or put an interesting look on your face. OK. Enough of that. Now look away a moment and be the person who you are when you're not looking in the mirror. Let your face lapse into your "default mode," the face you have when you're driving, for instance. Now, look back into the mirror without making adjustments. This is your portrayal of who you are to the world. Now smile. This is you on positive thoughts. Now laugh. This is you without stress. Who would you like to be? Which of the three would you like to meet? As we age, gravity works on our faces and what we consider a neutral face is actually easily interpreted as angry or sad or standoffish. Television people know this well and maintain a face that feels like a slight smile in order to look neutral. All we can do, short of expensive surgery, is to present a more positive facial invitation to those we come in contact with.

2. Keep track for several days of when you laugh, not just smile or make a short noise. We're talking *laugh* here, if only for several seconds. Make a goal to increase that by a small amount, say one more time than the usual. Seek out the situations or people who make you laugh. Avoid situations or people that make you feel sad, or angry, or bad about yourself. Consider them toxic, because indeed they are.

3. If you find you have not increased you laughter for a particular day, just laugh. "Fake it till you make it," as they say. Even forced laughter is beneficial.

4. Like Norman Cousins, find movies or TV shows that make you laugh. We're talking big, belly, milk-out-your-nose laughs. At least that should be the goal. Anything less is helpful and lays the groundwork for a lower threshold for laughing. Seek out comedians who do it for you. Kids. Kids laugh often and well. Spend some time with kids and you'll be laughing right along with them. Or find a "laughter yoga" class in your area. These classes are not so much about

stretching your muscles as they are about your ability to find your inner jovial self.

5. Spend time with friends, unless, of course, they're the Debbie Downer types. We laugh more when we're with others rather than alone or with our families. Seek out new activities with friends that provoke laughter: karaoke, comedy clubs, games, amusement parks, whatever brings out the kid in you.

6. Make a mental note every time you laugh: "I'm getting healthier. I'm going to do more of this." When you awake in the morning, and when you retire at night, make a mental list (or write it out if you are an engineer or accountant) of all you are grateful for in this day. This will help you focus on those positive things in your life rather than those that make you feel sorry for yourself. Remember, life's a head game. You choose happiness, laughter, joy, or you don't. You choose health, or you don't. You choose to age more successfully— or you don't.

IN A NUTSHELL

Do or do not. There is no try.

—YODA

You've made it through the Ten Tips to Achieve Authentic Health and Successful Aging. Now what?

Stick with your commitment to live a lifestyle that will build authentic health and the resilience necessary to navigate through the next phase of your life. Avoid setting expectations that are too ambitious; when you don't achieve them, you'll derail your momentum. Remember, there is no goal too small. Remember, also, that you must be the warrior for your own health and aging. It is whole-person strength—building physical, mental, social, and spiritual power—that will give you the authentic health and resilience you need. And lastly, never underestimate the ravages of the Big Uneasy, the damaging effects of self-induced chronic stress in your life.

Aging successfully is about avoiding or preventing occurrence of a disease or condition whenever possible, *or* identifying it early to prevent it from taking hold, *or*, if it does become established, limiting its negative effects. Beating yourself up about the fact that you do have the condition is useless and destructive to your efforts to keep growing.

If you're someone who wants the short version of everything, a cheat sheet, then here it is for the Ten Tips:

Move every day as part of your day, rather than as a scheduled event you can forgo if you get busy. Better to enjoy whatever type of movement you do. Better to move with someone else.

Learn something new every day. It can be a simple fact, or part of larger undertaking, like a language or a new craft, but seek out some new knowledge as part of your day.

Reach out to someone every day. It can be a smile to a cashier, or a nod to someone on the street, or reconnecting with people once important in your life. Whatever it is, welcome people into your life. Get rid of those defense mechanisms you developed in junior high, and be open to others.

Do something that scares you every day. It doesn't have to be bungee jumping (although if that is what you have always dreamed of doing, why not?), but it should be something that takes you out of your comfort zone, like traveling without reservations, or reaching out to new people.

Find something that will quiet your chattering mind if only for a few minutes each day. You'll know it when you find it. It will bring you peace and joy.

Find your purpose, the essence of your journey here on earth, and the reason to be grateful for this grand gift of life.

And above all, realize that life has surprises in store for you, some of which will require resilience. Find a lifestyle that encourages, nourishes, and builds whole-person strength, the warrior within you; a lifestyle that will connect you on a deep level with your core human needs and brings you authentic health; a lifestyle that will be as a symphony, bringing all those core components together as a masterpiece. The rest of your life depends on it.

And then, I met Alicia

Just as I was finalizing this manuscript, I attended the wedding of my friend Rick's son Heath. My friendship with Rick was forged in Germany decades ago as squadron mates flying F15s. At this magnificent California wedding, I observed a woman, perhaps in her eighties, interacting with the guests with a warm serene smile, and a nobility and grace that was frankly spellbinding. I made one of those decisions that change your life—I introduced myself to her. And it changed everything.

Alicia is Rick's aunt, and her story is one that's difficult to comprehend. Difficult because it is intensely painful if you make any attempt to place yourself in her shoes. Difficult because it portrays humans at the absolute boundaries of possibilities—their very best and their very worst. And difficult because it challenges all who hear it to question whether they could survive such devastating events with their humanity intact, indeed whether they could survive at all. Even as I write this, I'm struggling because my words are pale communicators of the reality of Alicia's story and because I'm overwhelmed with a sense of responsibility to do justice to this human drama. But here goes . . .

Alicia is nearly ninety, a vibrant, engaged, serene soul who observes the world with an expression of nurturing understanding and appreciative wonder. The wonder for me is with the journey she made to get to this day, to this conversation with me.

She was born in Poland, and as a young Jewish teenager in Poland, in 1940, her world came crashing down with the arrival of the Nazis in her small town. They quickly levied oppressive restrictions on the entire community and soon her father was arrested and disappeared forever from her life. Alicia and her sister fled the town and were able to live in another small town where there were no Germans but severe food shortages. They sold all they had for food. With the arrival of the Nazis to the new town, they were placed in a ghetto but survived on their wits and ability to understand German. It was here that Alicia discovered that Jews were being exterminated and she resolved to survive.

Soon she and her sister were sent to the Krakow ghetto and one day, while walking down a street, they were seized and transported to the infamous Auschwitz. "Worse than hell," this concentration camp was the scene of incomprehensible suffering and inhumanity. Alicia was tattooed, her head was shaved, and she was given dirty clothing to wear. From the very beginning, she knew she must be both clever and strong. Those who were weaker, who cried, or gave up, soon disappeared. She personally witnessed hundreds being taken to the crematorium and often saw many lined up outside the crematorium awaiting their turn. She remembers one night when all the Gypsies, hundreds, disappeared.

Because she knew German, Alicia was able to get work as a secretary, and although always hungry, she was able to get blankets and occasional news from the head of the warehouse. In June of 1944 she inwardly rejoiced to hear that the Allies had invaded Normandy. She had to hang on.

Her resolve was tested when she was caught while getting news and sent to solitary in a dungeon for eighteen days. She refused to cry or show any weakness and she believes this saved her. After solitary, as further punishment, she had to work hard labor and was soon sent to another camp in Germany where she worked in a munitions factory. Conditions there were horrid, with very hard work and even less food. Alicia admits she would not have survived much longer if the Americans had not freed her on April 18, 1945.

At this point in her story, Alicia paused. "The will to survive is very strong. If I were given a choice to be a beggar all my life or die, I would be a beggar because there would always be a little hope. The will to survive can also turn some into animals," she added, "doing whatever it takes to survive, even the most inhumane things." She breathed deeply. "I refused to do that."

With the war over, Alicia settled in a German town with her sister and began working for an organization helping the thousands of postwar refugees. She held on tightly to the possibility of emigrating to America. Her sister had been badly weakened by imprisonment, suffering from many diseases, but Alicia had remained well. "I don't know why," she says. Even through the lowest points, she had maintained a semblance of humor, joking about the guards' incompetence when they were forced to stand in line for hours while the guards attempted to count the prisoners.

Alicia was now hungry to learn. "I was curious and wanted to know about the universe, history, the human body, psychology, and how I was able to survive and maintain my humanity." She enrolled in a university. "I had no idea of where my family was, but the university opened a new world." She learned Russian in order to read Pushkin.

She and her sister eventually emigrated. Alicia had no difficulty adjusting to life in the United States because it is a "welcoming country, and I was never hungry." Alicia learned English, married a chemist, and had two girls. She embraced motherhood "with my whole heart." "I raised my girls in a morally rich environment," she says. "We lived modestly." Although they could not afford piano lessons, her husband taught both girls to play. Her daughters, like she and her husband, embraced learning, attended Ivy League colleges, and became prominent professionals.

The last ten years have once again challenged Alicia's resiliency. Her husband became forgetful and gradually lost his cognitive faculties. The last two years of his life, he was unable to speak. Alicia was committed to keeping him at home even at great emotional cost. "I had to watch this great brain and person rapidly decline." She recently lost him and felt she didn't have the strength to attend the funeral, but, of course, she did. "I had to pull myself together."

When asked what she would tell others about life and aging, she was quietly eloquent. "I lived from minute to minute and never lost my love of life. Life is sweet, the world a beautiful place with space for all of us. What does it matter what religion or nationality one has? People are people. Why should we have wars? Being a good person, doing no harm, is what matters." She adds, "I advise all not to live with a small horizon. Open your eyes and ears. There's so much to learn, so much friendship to have, so many opportunities to better ourselves. A positive outlook is key. I look at people with sad faces and feel sorry for them. Enjoy whatever is."

Alicia had nightmares for many years after the war. She felt she had to do something and so she connected with a former friend in Krakow and visited her. She went directly to the street where she was arrested. "No one chased me." She no longer had nightmares after that visit.

And so Alicia—witness to some of history's worst suffering, to atrocious inhumanity; a survivor, who suffered, and lost her home, her family, and then her beloved sister, and her revered husband—has some last words for me. "I believe in mankind."

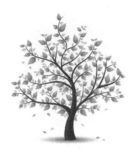

PART III

WHERE DO WE GO FROM HERE?

Come, my friends,
'Tis not too late to seek a newer world. . . .
Though much is taken, much abides; and though
We are not now that strength which in the old days
Moved earth and heaven, that which we are, we are,
One equal temper of heroic hearts,
Made weak by time and fate, but strong in will
To strive, to seek, to find, and not to yield.

—ALFRED, LORD TENNYSON, "ULYSSES"

CHAPTER 16

A LOOK INTO OUR FUTURE:
IT WON'T BE WHAT YOU THINK

We do not think ourselves into new ways of living,
we live ourselves into new ways of thinking.
—FRANCISCAN PRIEST
RICHARD ROHR, O.F.M.

The present is pregnant with the future.
—VOLTAIRE

Let's return to Dr. Ken Dychtwald, the author of *Age Wave*, whom we quoted in part I. He told us of the profound changes that will occur in our society as the wave of baby boomers turns sixty-five, as they will now at a rate of over eight thousand a day for the next seventeen years. He told us that older adults have been removed from their historical position of esteem and power, but only in the last couple of centuries. He continues in *Age Power*: "But they are not down for the count: If you look around, you'll notice that during the past several decades the elderly have multiplied, growing stronger, richer, and politically tougher. They are returning to the status and control that once was theirs."[1]

Older people will reclaim their previously held control, driven by the demographics and financial power. This is not, however, in my opinion, a formula for a positive evolution of our society. If you are young, it will be easy to resent a segment of the population that you support with your rising taxes (especially when you feel you will never be the beneficiary of similar support), that has the political and financial power, and that dominates the national policy debate. Intergenerational strife is inevitable under this scenario.

What is needed is a *shift in responsibility more than in power*, a shift that is the inevitable result not of demographics and financial dominance but of a recognition on the part of the greater society of the huge untapped treasure of human capital awaiting engagement: the experiential power, wisdom, and tempered passion for a higher purpose, and, on the part of older adults of their duty to continue to contribute for the betterment of that society. What we need, in fact, is Dr. Bill Thomas's concept of "Eldertopia." In a 2011 article in AARP International's *The Journal*, he defined Eldertopia as

> a community that improves the quality of life for people of all ages by strengthening and improving the means by which (1) the community protects, sustains, and nurtures its elders, and (2) the elders contribute to the well-being and foresight of the community. An Eldertopia that is blessed with a large number of older people is acknowledged to be "elder-rich" and uses this wealth to advance the good of all.[2]

Indeed, as the old begin to rise in influence, intergenerational strife can be avoided only if they don the cloak of the village elder, with a profound sense of responsibility for the entire group. Rather than promoting a self-serving, entitlement-minded approach to policy change, the old will once again have to assume the role of stewards of the common good. In his remarkable book, *From Age-ing to Sage-ing*, Zalman Schachter-Shalomi gives us a clear view of this revived role of the elder. Like Ken Dychtwald, he charts the marginalization of older adults beginning with the Industrial Revolution and continuing with the rapid technological and social change that has occurred since then. Schachter-Shalomi remains confident that we are about to enter a new period in which the elders will rise again to a restored state of relevance. He states, "I believe the time is coming when older people will convene councils of elders to share their dreams, meditations, and visions of a revived elderhood. As this happens, we will collectively dream the myths and create the models that will galvanize social change."[3]

David Gutmann has also been a consistent passionate voice for a return of elders as guides of culture. He writes, "We will have to enlist the elders, who have traditionally been the wardens of culture to help and guide us in . . . crafting the new myths on which reculturation can be based. We owe this redemption not only to our aging parents. We also owe it to the oncoming generations of children."[4]

The Elders

We're beginning to see examples of Gutmann's and Schachter-Shalomi's predictions even on a global scale. The Elders is an independent group of global leaders who no longer hold public office and who come together to use their influence and experience to address some of the most pressing problems facing the world today. Conceived by entrepreneur Richard Branson and musician Peter Gabriel, who both observed that some societies still looked to their elders for guidance, they wondered: In an increasingly interdependent world—a "global village"—could a group of respected elders provide guidance to solve global problems? They approached Nelson Mandela, who organized the effort and brought it to reality. So we wonder, isn't such an approach possible on a borough, town, city, regional, state, and national level? After all, it has only been a blink of a few generations in the long history of man that this has *not* been the case.

Our brave new old world

Empowered by the knowledge of what is possible, and what it takes to realize those possibilities, older adults will resist traditional paternalistic approaches to their needs and preferences. These new older adults will instead demand opportunities to continue to grow, to have purpose in their lives, and to remain engaged in society. Whether with paid work, volunteerism, or pro bono service, our new older adults will resist marginalization and seek to guide national, regional, and local policy beyond just the ballot box. Naturally more spiritual and appreciative of life and the human experience, they will seek out opportunities to make a difference, to guide younger generations, and to be the voice of reason and humanism in an ever more dangerous world. They will demand living arrangements that acknowledge and foster growth no matter what impairments might be present. These new older adults will also resist group characterization, *demanding recognition as individuals rather than as a demographic cohort.*

Even the language of aging will change with the cultural shift driven by an enlightened view of the potential associated with older adults. Terms and phrases pregnant with stereotypical baggage will have to go: *senior center, nursing home, retirement home, senior moment* (all ages have these moments), *over the hill, senior, the elderly,* and so many more. The media, who must assume responsibility for some of the marginalization of older adults, must now follow the lead of progressive companies like Dove, whose award-winning "Campaign for Real Beauty" abandoned the traditional view of older adults as either "broken adults" or super seniors in favor of a realistic view. One ad featured a ninety-five-year-old asking, "Withered or wonderful? Will society ever accept old can be beautiful?"[5]

As our society evolves and accommodates our older adults, significant benefits will accrue to both. Our national policy will be guided less by partisanship, greed, blind ambition, and prejudice and more by an appreciation of the benefit of a population approach to health, an inclusive view of the implications of any policy, and a long view of the advantages and disadvantages of any decisions. Older adults, on the other hand, will realize the benefits well articulated in the research on aging—having a sense of purpose, being engaged in life, continuing to build physical and mental abilities—and will consequently have less need for expensive healthcare and social services.

Let's fast-forward a decade or so and take a closer look at such a future in three basic areas. In this look, I have the added luxury of being a "lead boomer," and so have been able to provide a reality check to the predictions of other experts and futurists.

Where will they (we) live?

Freed of the tyranny of making where they live a visible statement of their success in life, no longer following blind youthful aspirations of larger or even multiple houses or of curb appeal, and having moved beyond, for the most part, the need to accommodate large numbers of visiting family or friends, our older adults of the near future will use more functional criteria in choosing where they live. As with many older adults of today, they will want to free themselves of the burden of maintenance and upkeep and will seek out areas that offer opportunities for them to pursue or continue pastimes they enjoy or have always wanted to try. Weather will remain a factor. They will also want to be less isolated than they most likely had become over the years in their previous house, looking instead for opportunities to meet like-minded peers. They will travel more and will therefore choose to live reasonably close to airports. And of course, they will ensure that quality healthcare is available, just in case.

So far, that doesn't sound much different from what most older adults of today might list as their criteria for where they will live. The difference is that *the choices will be made with more purpose.* Indeed, knowing that these choices are much more significant for how they age, how independent they will remain, and the overall quality of their aging experience, our new older adults will move beyond the mere criteria of recreation, beyond long-held views of what retirement should be, and beyond the recommendations of friends and family. They will instead seek out opportunities for meaningful friendships and social connection: connection that enhances rather than diminishes the number and quality of social experiences, that involves people of all ages, including young adults and children, and that enhances their knowledge of the world and builds genuine compassion and sense of community.

Our new older adult will be drawn to a living situation that stimulates physical activity. We are all influenced by our surroundings, and those where the culture is one of movement—walking, biking, swimming, adventure travel, volleyball, yoga, fitness classes—will be of paramount importance to the older adults of the new future. Even when there are physical issues, an environment where possibilities and accommodation for such issues is the focus will help older adults flourish.

Our new older adults will want to be surrounded by opportunities to learn new things. Much as it is at a university (indeed, a university, where growing is the currency, is an excellent model for the successful older adult community of the future), the norm will be to discover and grow. Stagnation, rigidity, prejudice, and the exclusion of new ideas, technologies, and opinions will not thrive in the successful community of the new older adult. The self-imposed caricature of the older adult with negative overtones will fade as more people understand the deleterious effects of such deprecating dialogue, and as peers become less tolerant of it.

Lastly, the living situation of enlightened older adults will stimulate and offer robust opportunity for meaningful living and purpose. Whether through the influence of their peers or acknowledgment on the part of the greater community that older adults are a powerful resource, our successfully aging older adults will be surrounded with a milieu of personal responsibility, accountability, and respect for their status. Like village elders of the past, older adults living in such an environment will be sought out for their valuable solutions to the society's challenges. It will matter less whether these characteristics are in retirement communities, NORCs (naturally occurring retirement communities), or in subsets of the greater community. It will be the culture of social connection and growth that matters most.

What will they (we) do?

Our emerging, enlightened older adults will evolve out of the recreation, entitlement, or self-absorption stereotype and will look to characterize this phase of their lives with purposeful engagement. Their hours will be spent seeking growth, whether physically, mentally, socially, or spiritually. Some of their activities will appear to be unchanged from those of today's older adults, yet they will differ because they will be chosen for specific reasons, for the specific benefits they offer to our new older adults' aging experience, and for their contribution to overall successful aging. Many will elect to continue to work for pay, but more and more this choice will reflect a conscious decision to contribute or find purpose beyond the financial compensation.

Social connection will be fun, yes. It will fill otherwise lonely hours, but most importantly, it will enhance brain and immune function, and make decline less likely. Physical movement will also increase the likelihood of remaining independent longer. Our new older adults will want opportunities to grow intellectually. The meaning of lifelong learning will expand beyond classes at the local college to new skills: in music, language, writing, art, woodworking, understanding diversity, teaching, mentoring, and educational travel. A community where this is the norm rather than the exception will be attractive to our new older adults, who realize that the brain is a magnificent untapped resource. Time spent helping other living things in their journey through life will offer satisfaction, as always, but our enlightened older adults will also realize that the quality, and perhaps even quantity, of their own lives will be enriched.

What will they (we) buy?

I cannot speculate specifically on how the successful aging-savvy older adults will spend their money; however, it is clear from the above descriptions of where they will choose to live and spend their time that they will seek and value *experience*. Whether it's an opportunity to grow physically, mentally, socially, or spiritually, the value of resources to enhance such growth will rise. Rather than looking for bragging rights, or pursuing unexamined desires of their younger years, our enlightened older adult will seek out those commodities that will help them to become all they can be, that help them satisfy core needs for a meaningful life as defined not by the media, or advertising, or ambition, or stereotypical views of what older adults want, but by an honest look into what it means to be authentic in older age, and by a knowledge of what it takes to age successfully.

A tipping point

Malcolm Gladwell, in his thought-provoking 2000 book *The Tipping Point*, writes of epidemics of change: "Ideas and products and messages and behaviors spread just like viruses do."[6] Gladwell goes on: "We need to prepare ourselves for the possibility that sometimes big changes follow from small events, and that sometimes these changes can happen very quickly." Sudden change is the basis for his ideas on the "tipping point," which is "the moment of critical mass, the threshold, the boiling point."

Katie Sloan, in addition to holding several leadership positions at the International Association of Homes and Services for the Aging, is chief operations officer and senior vice president of LeadingAge, an organization whose members are not-for-profit retirement communities. In addressing retirement-living executives about the future, Sloan threw down the gauntlet and challenged the industry to be prepared for a new older adult: "There is an attitudinal fault line around shifting expectations. We need to listen hard and actively because what we learn will define our success in future years."[7] Fault line indeed, for the demographic pressure is rising and it will let go with cataclysmic results.

Although the aging of the nation has, of course, occurred gradually, the response to it will not. The societal shift, more a cultural shift, is, I believe, imminent. Rising healthcare costs associated with chronic disease and aging, the financial challenges facing the nation, the growing awareness that much more is possible as we age, the "retirement" of the lead boomers, a growing disenchantment with an acquisition approach to happiness and fulfillment, the accelerating divisive and mean-spirited public discourse—all this and more has created the perfect storm for a dramatic shift in how we as a society view, appreciate, and incorporate older adults. The conditions for dramatic change as articulated by Gladwell are at hand. The *stickiness*—i.e., the notion that the change has the ability to attract attention—is there, I believe, in the idea that we all can age in a better way, slowing decline and living a life characterized more by growth and purpose than by loss. The *context*—i.e., the situation that favors the change—is clearly present, with an aging society facing an oppressive burden of chronic disease, and the failure of the postindustrial period to improve all of society. These conditions are, I believe, about to spark an eruption within our society that will turn our world upside down: older adults will no longer be the problem but will be part of the solution; being old will give a person a revered status; the focus of media, marketing, and policy will be more inclusive of older adults.

Some will be positioned to accept this shift and will thrive. Providers of services attractive to growth-hungry, engaged, health- and independence-minded older adults will flourish. More traditional, intractable, ageism-infected organizations will wither. Senior-living providers poised to become destinations for individual growth will explode. Those rooted in nursing-home, paternalistic, and medical-model approaches will be doomed. Senior centers that become centers for healthy, successful aging will survive. Those unable to evolve beyond an entertainment, "keep busy" approach will disappear. Those who sell products that enhance experience, providing opportunities to grow physically, mentally, socially, and spiritually, will succeed. Those that focus on the response to decline will not. We can already see minor adjustments toward a paradigm shift in the media: more older adults in ads, portrayed as active and engaged, more older adults as pundits on talk shows. Such adjustments are the bell cows of a coming stampede.

What can we expect?

As Dychtwald's "Age Wave" approaches, older adults will be more visible. They will also be . . .

- more abundant
- healthier
- more active
- more engaged (work, volunteerism, activism)
- more targeted by media
- more politically active
- more powerful (richer, more outspoken)
- living in mainstream communities rather than retirement communities

Older adults will be more valued . . .
- for the above reasons
- as mentors (a return to the elder as consultant)
- as consumers
- as national-policy contributors

Older adults will seek . . .
- serious roles in society
- multigenerational contact
- significant social engagement
- opportunities to learn
- opportunities to grow

Older adults will resist . . .
- ageism of any form—subtle or overt
- language and terms associated with a decline-only concept of aging
- marginalization within society (in politics, healthcare, the professional field, and media)
- all traditional stereotypes of aging
- group characterization
- pandering

CHAPTER 17

A MORAL IMPERATIVE: WHEN THERE'S REALLY NO CHOICE

Those that have the privilege to know,
have the duty to act.
—ALBERT EINSTEIN

Whenever I'm struggling with a new initiative and getting pessimistic about whether we can pull it off, my friend and colleague Dave Gobble smiles and says, "Four-minute mile, Roger," and just like that, I'm focused on the solution again. Prior to 1954, no one had run a mile in less than four minutes. In fact, esteemed physiologists went on record to say it was not possible for a human to do such a thing. In that year, Roger Bannister ran a mile in 3:59.4. Two months later another runner broke the four-minute barrier. Today, high school students have run the mile in less than four minutes. In fact, the fastest time is currently around 3:43, a full seventeen seconds off the supposed four-minute barrier!

Much too often, barriers to our own growth are self-imposed. It's comfortable to ascribe our limitations, or our unwillingness to attempt growth, to impossibility. The parents of adolescents know this mind-set all too well. We know this. When we are forced to confront the reality that something is indeed possible, we are also forced out of our comfort zone. We grow, or we don't. As Yoda says, we do or we don't do. There is no try.

So, now the cat's out of the bag. We know that how we age depends primarily on us, on our lifestyles, on the choices we make every day. We know that so much more is possible as we age. We know we can continue to grow no matter what life deals us. We know that the four-minute mile of aging was a culturally imposed barrier built by low expectations, forced disengagement, loss of reverence, low societal value, and overall ignorance. The barrier has been smashed by the MacArthur Study and two decades of subsequent research. Much of the decline associated with aging can be prevented. Much of the burden of an aging society can be avoided. It's not only possible, but it has been repeatedly demonstrated.[1]

Our own goal with Masterpiece Living—of actualizing the research findings and providing tools and environments to assist older adults in modifying and refining their lifestyles in order to age in a better way—has been realized and is growing more powerful with each refinement, with each new community partner, with each new analysis of our data. A true *movement* is under way. The four-minute barrier of ageism, complacency, ignorance, and paternalism is fraying. Yet we have only scratched the surface. Taking the next step toward an enlightened approach to aging and a national policy on aging will not be as easy as breaking the four-minute barrier. Often the barriers are perched on very high ground—moral high ground.

Caring as barrier

The senior-living industry provides us with a powerful example of lofty barriers. In the late nineteenth century, at the height of the Industrial Revolution, many older Americans, having been transplanted to the city for work, now lacked the social support structure they had previously found in their villages and towns. If the husband were to die, the widow was often immediately destitute, homeless, and penniless. Religious and charitable organizations, seeing the need, founded almshouses, or poorhouses. These were not desirable places to end up, yet they grew with the growing need. The Social Security Act of 1935 helped evolve these almshouses into senior-living businesses, since now many residents had some ability to pay. The Medicare Act of 1965 further changed senior living into what we see today.

Whether it is a continuing-care retirement community (CCRC), assisted living, or skilled nursing, providers of senior living today are experts at providing care. For almost a century, these institutions have been taking care of the destitute and then of the aging with impairments, and they've developed reputations as both caring organizations and experts in delivering care. When someone is in need, when someone is impaired, or sick, or infirm, they look to these organizations as places to live. CCRCs have, in fact, had difficulty getting older adults to move into the independent-living parts of their communities, because many of those who are still functioning well "aren't ready yet" for the traditional caring services these communities are most famous for.

Despite this now incorrect popular assessment of what many senior-living communities provide, most of these communities have done relatively little to wander from their tried-and-true reputation of delivering excellent care. They have started wellness programs that go not much further than an exercise room and the donated equipment. They even speak about a "holistic" approach to wellness, but other than this rhetoric and a few anecdotes involving one or two exceptional individual residents, they have done the minimum needed to compete for the new older adult seeking more from a living situation, seeking more than care. Despite a growing realization that new older adults are aware of the research on aging, on brain fitness, on the importance of socialization and purpose, and consequently are demanding more, these communities remain timid, unwilling to leave the safe bank of their reputation for caring, fearful of reinventing themselves. After all, isn't quality care and nurturing a fine reputation to have?

It is, of course, but the world of aging has shifted to a new orbit and it will get very empty and lonely up on the moral high ground of caring as a more savvy group of older adults is drawn to places that promise continued growth—physical, mental, social, and spiritual. Places that are what Larry Minnix—president and CEO of LeadingAge, an association of not-for-profit organizations that is dedicated to making America a better place to grow old—calls "Centers for Healthy Aging." I like to call such places "Destinations for Successful Aging." Communities in our Masterpiece Living Network who attain the highest levels of culture enrichment are designated as "Centers for Successful Aging."

And there are other reasons, also camped out on the moral high ground, that some offer for not making the transition to growth in senior living. Minimizing risk is one. This objections sounds like this: "They could fall." "Regulations prevent us from offering challenging programming." "We do not want to create unreasonable expectations." "It's not what *our* residents want. They are happy with things as they are." "We've tried that." "We're already doing that." Yet all these melt under scrutiny. Falls are in fact reduced when someone is moving more and becoming more confident in his abilities. Regulations, in fact, call for senior-living communities to provide environments that help residents "attain the highest practicable physical, mental, and psychosocial well-being."[2]

It's a shame. For the most part, providers of senior living are a highly dedicated and altruistic group. They are wired to do the right thing. But, unable to evolve beyond the gold standard of caring to the platinum standard of continued growth and successful aging, they are struggling for relevance. Dr. Joseph Coughlin is director of the Massachusetts Institute of Technology AgeLab, whose mission is to invent new ideas and creatively translate technologies into practical solutions that improve people's health and enable them to "do things" throughout their lifespan. In a 2011 summary of a strategy session sponsored by the International Council on Active Aging,[3] Dr. Coughlin concluded that

- Senior living must change.
- Change will not come from within.
- There must be a new business model.
- The "aging in place" preference will create a whole new area of business.
- The new older adult will want customized services.

In light of the latest research on aging, the right thing—the moral imperative—is to facilitate and assist older adults in continuing to grow. Provide care where needed, yes, but not as the primary service, but as a necessary part of coaching aging adults, even significantly impaired older adults, to be all they can be. I believe that the change will come from outside the field, from objective problem solvers unencumbered by traditions of caring. However, I also believe that the change must involve experts from senior living. Fortunately, there are visionary communities that are making the transition and will hopefully lead most of their colleagues to a new model for senior living that better serves the new older adult.

Evolution is occurring and will continue to occur within the medical field. With healthcare costs looming like a time bomb and threatening the financial foundation of our country, healthcare legislation is providing, and will surely continue to provide, partial solutions by incentivizing a more preventive approach rather than a disease-based, fee-for-service model of care. And why shouldn't this happen? Take, for instance, falls in older adults. In 2000, the total direct medical costs of all fall injuries for people sixty-five and older exceeded $19 billion.[4] By 2020, the annual direct and indirect cost of fall injuries is expected to reach $54.9 billion.[5] In a 2002 study, Medicare costs per fall averaged between $9,113 and $13,507.[6] Yet we know that something as simple as a home exercise program can reduce falls and injuries by as much as 35 percent.[7]

Medical care providers will take a closer look at what it takes to get, be, and remain healthy while aging. Much like the oil companies that are beginning to see themselves as energy companies, the medical industry will begin to view itself as a true *health* industry rather than just a curing or caring industry. It too will be looking for ways to meet the full range of health and successful-aging needs of all. Organizations and communities that approach aging and chronic conditions with a true holistic approach, one based on our core needs as humans, will be attractive as partners to both older adults and medical providers and insurers. This environment will provide an exciting opportunity for senior-living communities to reach out to the greater community to offer their expertise on successful aging.

One of our more progressive partners, Sun Health in Phoenix, is doing just that, reaching out to the aging west Phoenix area to provide its successful-aging expertise in order to help those who choose to live in their homes remain as independent as possible for as long as possible. Their Masterpiece Living–fueled, holistic approach and their expertise in building environments that foster growth is breaking down walls between the retirement community and the greater community it is part of. The winners of this enlightened approach will be the residents of west Phoenix, medical providers and insurers, the residents of the retirement community, and Sun Health itself. Again, it is the acknowledgment and incentivization of what it takes to be authentically healthy and to age successfully that makes this approach a much more cost-effective and, frankly, morally correct way of addressing health and aging.

The right thing to do

So, once again, we're left with the knowledge that we can age in a better way. That given a few minor adjustments in the environment, some education, and a few tools, older adults can indeed increase the likelihood they will live long and die short. That we all, in fact, can enjoy a much higher quality of life and avoid much of the painful and expensive decline often seen in the years, even decades, before death. How can we ignore this? How can we, as individuals, as organizations, or as a society, not use this knowledge to bring it to reality for all? Are we not, as Dr. Jonas Salk frequently stated, obligated to make the world a better place? To do what we can to better the human condition? This is indeed the definition of moral imperative: the obligation to make something happen because we know it is the right thing. When we knew that with the smallpox vaccine and a determined effort we could eradicate the disease from the planet, were we not obligated to proceed? Likewise with polio? When we discovered that secondhand smoke could cause cancer and lung disease, were we not compelled to protect nonsmokers?

Are we not as individuals, knowing that how we age depends on our lifestyle, obligated to decide whether we indeed want to be around for our grandchildren's weddings? To raise our children with the knowledge that their lifestyle has profound implications? To cease with a victim mentality and pursue continued growth no matter what life may have in store for us? Can we smoke, or gain large amounts of weight, or be sedentary, or avoid learning, and expect an aging experience other than decline? We all have a choice in how we will live our lives, but we cannot expect to live a high-risk lifestyle and be surprised when those risks take a huge chunk out of the quality and quantity of our lives.

Are we not as collections of people—schools, workplaces, towns, and cities—obligated to educate and provide environments where people are aware of their own potential to have a higher quality of life and avoid painful and expensive decline? How can we provide any service to people and ignore this very basic requirement for a better life? And these imperatives are not just for those in aging services. I believe the messages of lifestyle and authentic health and successful aging must begin in kindergarten. Anything less is tantamount to neglect.

As a society, isn't providing an environment where citizens can flourish, experience the highest quality of life, and be healthy a core function of government? There may be some who argue that it's the obligation of other organizations, but "life, liberty, and the pursuit of happiness" covers it for me. Not only is it advantageous for a society to have high-functioning, fulfilled, and engaged citizens, but with healthcare costs exponentially increasing and threatening the financial stability and strategic growth of the nation, doesn't it seem plausible that public policy should reflect a commitment to assist people in preventing disease and decline, and in continuing to be viable and engaged?

What if?

My grandson Dylan is an intelligent, inquiring nine-year-old. He showers me with "what if" questions, and I feel blessed. Some questions are outrageous yet show an unbounded creativity and fearless desire to expand the boundaries of his world. He quite naturally does what Seth Godin, the popular entrepreneurial advisor and author, calls "poking the box"[8]— in other words, he challenges the status quo. I wonder when I stopped asking "what if" questions. Was it the first time someone laughed at my question? Or when a teacher told me to get serious? Or when I tried one of the "what ifs" and it failed miserably? Whenever it was, it was a shame, and I'm back in the business as of now.

What if each person who actually accomplished his physician's top recommendation for improving his health got a tax break as well as a premium reduction from his insurance company? What if Social Security were slightly increased if the recipient volunteered for an approved organization that needed assistance? What if groups of older adults were assigned duties as event-planning consultants for schools, towns, cities, and other organizations? What if twentieth-century history classes in schools and universities required older adults who had lived through the time to contribute? What if colleges and universities were required to have a minimum percentage of their students be older adults in order to obtain financial support?

What if an appointed, term-limited, pro bono board of directors of older adults gave nonbinding guidance on all major national policy? What if a national resource of screened older adults provided day care to infants and children at a nominal fee? What if there were a national registry of experienced older adult professionals who provided consultation on issues within their field of expertise? What if every child wanting or requiring an older-adult friend and advisor could readily be connected with one? What if there were a national registry of volunteers to work on trails, hold premature infants in hospitals, teach skills to inner-city boys and girls, or perform any task a school, town, city, or state might have a need for? What if older adults were seen as the potential solution to many of the problems facing towns, cities, municipalities, states, and organizations? What if older adults were seen as a resource instead of a burden? What if older adults began taking the advice author Marc Freedman gives in his book *The Big Shift: Navigating the New Stage Beyond Midlife*⁹ and began to pursue meaningful work that improves society?

Of course, anyone can provide a list of reasons why these "what ifs" shouldn't happen. Creativity and brave new approaches are not without risks, but when the potential benefit of lowered healthcare costs for successfully aging older adults is huge, when the possible solution to multiple seemingly unsolvable societal problems are staring us in the face, when the potential for building a national community guided by humanistic values is readily available, is it not worth the risk? There are those who believe that the way any society treats its animals, children, and older adults defines that society. Is it not worth exploring at least the possibility that older adults have the potential to age in a way that significantly limits decline, that they are not a drain but a powerful resource for guidance, nurturing, expertise, and overall functional stability of our nation? What, in fact, do we have to lose in trying? I believe we risk nothing in exploring this possibility, and much by not trying.

CHAPTER 18

BRINGING "WHAT IF?" TO REALITY:
THE REST OF THE MASTERPIECE LIVING STORY

Knowing is not enough; we must apply.
Willing is not enough; we must do.

—GOETHE

The world we have created is a product of our
thinking. It cannot be changed without changing our
thinking.

—ALBERT EINSTEIN

In 1999, the Masterpiece Living development team, called the Healthy Aging Working Group—or the HAWGs—began a journey of discovery. We were enthusiastic about what was possible, and ignited by a vision of making that happen. What if we could help all older adults age more successfully? How could we make it the norm rather than the exception? What would it take?

We were a long way from that vision. We were facing a stereotype of aging that portrayed decline as the dominant possibility, a stereotype that focused on caring, comfort, and security with little consideration of growth and potential. We were facing an aging-services industry and a public policy that was based on this stereotype. The task loomed, daunting.

We luckily decided on a kaizen approach of our own. We would take it one small step at a time. As a starting point, we needed a way to help older adults take a look at their lifestyle and get feedback. We needed resources—tools, really—that older adults and those working with them could use to do this.

As much as possible, the tools we chose would have to be reasonably well established in order to provide us with "normative data" (what is normal in a similar population) with which we could compare our data. With Bob Kahn's guidance, we chose several of the tools used by the MacArthur Study and then modified them to create a Lifestyle Review. To assess physical status, we sought established but easily administered tools to develop a Mobility Review. Lastly, to assess risk, we called in Mayo Clinic to provide its newly developed Health Risk Assessment. These tools would allow us to take an inventory of an individual's current lifestyle as it related to aging successfully. Next, with the help of Katie Hammond, a doctoral candidate at the University of South Florida, we developed a feedback report that was both educational and, we hoped, motivational.

So, our initial approach was: (1) educate older adults on the research findings and what indeed was possible, (2) give them the opportunity to take the Lifestyle Inventory, (3) provide feedback, (4) discuss the feedback in a one-on-one or group session with a lifestyle coordinator, (5) foster empowerment with a true coaching relationship, and (6) repeat the Lifestyle Inventory in a year. Would it work? Would older adults be willing to take the Lifestyle Inventory? Would the feedback motivate them to make changes? Would the likelihood of their aging in a better way change over a year? After nearly two years of intermittent meetings and prolonged discussions, it was time to find out.

Will Masterpiece Living work?

Who were to be our first subjects? With the Westport Senior Living Fund, which my brother Larry managed, we had access to two continuing-care retirement communities in Florida. These were retirement communities that offered four levels of living: independent, assisted, skilled nursing, and memory care. We decided to initially concentrate on older adults living independently, although we were fully committed to bring Masterpiece Living to assisted living, skilled nursing, and the memory unit.

In the summer of 2001 we began the pilot study at both Florida communities with training of the staff and the education of a small group of resident leaders on the new research. We told the resident leaders about the importance of lifestyle on how we age, and how Masterpiece Living could assist them to age more successfully. After this period of education and training, we launched Masterpiece Living for a small cadre of volunteer residents, mostly resident leaders of various committees. We knew we were limiting the effect of Masterpiece Living in selecting this group. These were adventurous older adults, who as leaders within the community led lifestyles already similar in many areas to that which the MacArthur Study had found more commonly associated with success in aging. So, the "delta," the amount of change between the before and after, in risk and overall lifestyle, would be smaller with this group. However, we would need them to help motivate their less adventurous neighbors to participate when we expanded the initiative.

The desired outcome of the Lifestyle Inventory and feedback process was to create sophisticated consumers of the programming available at the community. Rather than participate in "activities" designed to keep people busy, an approach we considered paternalistic and reeking of ageism, these educated older adults would now know where they were at risk, whether in the physical, intellectual, social, or spiritual components of their lives, and would seek out programming that would lower their specific risks—i.e., "purposeful programming." These people would know what they needed and would seek it out.

"Stunning" results

As planned, we repeated the Lifestyle Inventory on the initial cadre after one year. The results were, as one member of the HAWGs remarked, "stunning." We saw significant reduction in the Mayo Health Risk Assessment–measured risks, both medical and lifestyle. We saw improvement in overall Mobility Review scores, which measured gait, balance, range of motion, and strength—all correlating strongly with lowered risk of falls. Mean self-rated health (how healthy we think we are), a strong indicator of how someone will age, was the same as that of a group *ten years younger*. We were cautiously elated.

The group all agreed that, despite the initial very positive findings, we should collect a third data point at two years to ensure that the findings were not a fluke. The two-year data, though in general not as dramatic as the first-year changes, were nonetheless strongly consistent with the findings of the MacArthur Study. We were lowering risks of decline.

With some measures we saw growth over a year; with others, we saw merely stability. Dr. Kahn quickly eliminated any disappointment some of us might have had. Stability in the ninth or ten decade of life, he reminded us, was *bordering on miraculous*. The MacArthur Study had been validated. Our applied approach had worked. Our next decisions would be critical to the future of the entire initiative.

Where to go from here?

With the data showing that the Masterpiece Living approach to the MacArthur research findings and successful aging was effective, Larry and I were ready to begin dissemination of the program. Prior to signing on with the HAWGs, Bob Kahn had extracted a promise from Larry: we would not disseminate until Bob thought we were ready. This was a critical and fortunate promise. Moving ahead at that point would have doomed the entire effort to the status of another holistic-wellness program. For it was what we learned in the next two years of piloting Masterpiece Living that ultimately defined it as a *movement* rather than a program, as a fundamental paradigm shift in our approach to aging. That defining piece of information was this: *Any effort to influence a person's lifestyle toward one that resulted in successful aging had the best results when it took place within the context of a facilitative culture—a culture that was devoid of ageism, a culture that believed that older adults could continue to grow throughout their lives, even with impairments.* Basically, where you hung your hat was key to your aging. If the place you lived functioned as a cheerleader for you, you flourished.

We were indeed moving toward the conclusion that culture was an important ingredient, perhaps the key ingredient. We were considering developing training for all who worked in the community. This training would address what was possible in aging and change, and what role each staff member had in helping residents age more successfully. But it was Tim Parker, the executive director of University Village, our very first Masterpiece Living community, who showed us just how important culture was.

Tim makes it cultural

Tim challenged his directors, all of his directors—in dining, maintenance, accounting, transportation, housekeeping, and every other department in the retirement community—to bring something more to the community. He challenged them to look at the skills, hobbies, and interests of those working in their department (including themselves) and decide what they would offer the residents of University Village beyond their assigned responsibilities. Tim had each department present its offerings at a town meeting, and the residents voted on the most appealing. From that point on, the directors and their departments would be responsible for providing the promised offerings. And that's what happened. The director of maintenance offered, then led, offsite nature walks. The human resources director led a current-events discussion session, and the director of accounting taught casino gambling!

Tim's challenge was immensely successful. First of all, it made for an engaging, community-wide event, bringing more of the residents out of their apartments and to the town meeting. It engaged staff members in a way they had never been before. Staff members later related how much they enjoyed the enhanced role. In fact, when the director of human resources had to move back to his home state to tend to family problems, he publicly stated that the part of his time at University Village he would miss most was his current-affairs sessions with the residents. He said he never would have interacted with residents had it not been for those sessions.

The result of Tim's challenge, which was particularly informative for our group, was an obvious shift in the overall environment at University Village. That single revelation brought the word *culture* to life for both residents and staff. The place became a hotbed of learning, change, and growth. Staff members, as well as residents, welcomed the change. No longer was there departmental isolation—the silo effect—from the real mission of University Village. All were now working to make it place where all would grow.

Culture was no longer an abstract concept, no longer a pie-in-the-sky goal to enhance successful aging. It became a tangible, visible characteristic of the community. Culture was not just about leadership and the lifestyles department talking about successful aging. It was *everyone* believing that they had a role in that culture. And that culture was about growth. Growth for all, no matter what their age or impairment. This culture says, "OK. You're here. What do you want to do with the rest of your life? What is it that you have always wanted to do? What is your purpose? Can we (all in this community) assist you in any way? What are you going to add to this community?" These questions are not only stimulants to successful aging and higher quality of life; they're reminiscent, in an anthropological way, of the kind of environment in which we lived and thrived for most of the time we humans have been on earth. It's not that these kinds of questions were asked; it's that the answers were self-evident in these ancestral tribes and villages.

Laying the foundation

After a third year of pilot data was in, it was clear we were still on the right road. Risks were dropping. Mobility was improving. Lifestyles were leaning more toward the recommended lifestyles for successful aging. Resident data for our pilot population was still comparable to that of people ten years younger. Testimonies from older adults were pouring in. At this point, however, we were no more than a research-based, super-wellness program. We talked about culture change, and Tim's challenge at University Village gave us a glimpse of what it could be, but we offered little to help a community culture evolve into one of growth. It was time to move out from the rest of the wellness pack. Our next step was to enrich the environments where older adults were attempting to modify their lifestyles.

We spent the next three years developing tools and resources to help a community evolve its culture from one where comfort and security were the defining characteristics to one where growth was the currency, from a culture that provided what a zoo does for its residents to one that provided what a university does for its students: a culture where physical, intellectual, social, and spiritual growth is expected, nurtured, and facilitated. This brought us into new territory, where *every* staff member in the community had a role in culture; where the environment moved from a cruise ship–entertainment approach to one of growth; from a medical, paternalistic, "We'll help you when you get sick" model, to an approach of "Tell us how we can help you be all you can be." As you saw in part I of this book, we, in fact, were not inventing a new culture, but were dusting off a few hundred years' worth of dust from one that we humans had been living in for eons. We were, as in the 1985 movie, going *back to the future*.

Showtime

We were chomping at the bit to begin dissemination of Masterpiece Living, but we believed these extra culture-focused efforts would pay off, would define us, would help us achieve our mission to maximize the unique human potential of older adults and build environments where this was more likely to happen. We were correct.

In the spring of 2007, we were ready. We added Emily Parker (now Emily Warren) to our full-time staff of one (that would be me). A remarkably talented young Canadian woman with a passion for helping older adults, she came from a family familiar with the aging-services industry. Our team could have been characterized by Shakespeare's words from *A Midsummer Night's Dream*: "Though she be but little, she is fierce." Fired by our data and passion for making a difference, and still without sales or marketing expertise, we launched into disseminating Masterpiece Living into the world of continuing-care retirement communities. A partnership with Ziegler, a formidable force in the senior living, gave us enhanced credibility in our discussions with potential new partners.

The task of defining who we were and what we were attempting to do was daunting. In a profession with over a century of tradition of providing care, comfort, and security, the idea of facilitating growth was novel. Since aging services were primarily focused on caring for older adults, conservatism and healthy skepticism were understandably a major part of the culture. Once, however, early adopters like American Baptist Homes of the West were willing to give Masterpiece Living a try, we were on our way. And as they began to show similar outcomes to those shown in our pilot data, the task became easier. Today we are able to articulate more clearly who we are and what Masterpiece Living is.

Masterpiece Living is both *who we are* and *what we provide*. We are a multi-specialty group with a vision of maximizing the potential of all older adults. Our strategy to achieve this vision is threefold:

- We empower older adults to take control of their own aging.

- We help transform communities of all kinds into centers for aging successfully—places where older adults will continue to grow.

- We are committed to influencing a public policy that acknowledges that all older adults have potential, can continue to grow, and are a valuable resource for societies.

Our tactics are to . . .

- provide tools to empower older adults to adopt lifestyles known to result in a better aging experience
- partner with communities to provide environments for older adults that foster growth, engagement, and purposeful living
- track outcomes in order to build compelling cases for a more enlightened aging policy

We provide . . .

- a *partnership* dedicated to making communities attractive to older adults who wish to be all they can be
- a *respected team* of multi-specialty consultants
- an ever-growing array of *highly effective deliverables* to educate, train, coach, track outcomes, and articulate success within the community

Looking back, looking ahead

We have enjoyed robust growth within the senior-living industry, but even more rewarding is the intense interest, of late, in a better way to age from other sectors, such as senior centers, towns and cities, healthcare providers and insurers both private and government, and older adults living in their homes and wishing to stay vital and engaged longer than their grandparents and parents did. We relish working with these groups, for we know it's the way to our ultimate goal of influencing a more enlightened public policy on aging. Clearly, expanding within senior living is an important goal for us, for we feel strongly that whatever public policy lies ahead to address an aging nation, the talented and dedicated people within aging services will play a major role.

However, it will be the application of what we have learned in our 15-year journey with our senior living partners, to our new initiative—Masterpiece Life–which will reach out to people living in the greater community, providing us with the power of numbers to effect policy change. We relish the challenge of using technology to connect with people who remain in their cherished homes, and helping them to age in a better way.

Our potential influence on public policy was dramatically improved when, in 2012, the MacArthur Foundation awarded our joint proposal with the University of Michigan a grant to bring Masterpiece Living to affordable housing. With Drs. Toni Antonucci and Bob Kahn leading the effort, we have successfully introduced successful aging into three affordable-housing communities owned by our very first partners, American Baptist Homes of the West. We are very pleased with the outcomes in this very important initiative and look forward to expanding this effort.

Also exciting was the 2012 addition of our first senior center partner, Four Pointes Center for Successful Aging in Grand Haven, Michigan. Brigit Hassig and her team of talented and passionate people began a national movement to bring successful aging to all. They have seen spectacular increases in engagement in her growing population. Masterpiece Living made a major step toward bringing environments of growth to reality when, in the Fall of 2013, it debuted a major innovation with the Guidelines to Become a Certified Center for Successful Aging. These guidelines provided criteria and a roadmap for any community to "bring it to the next level," (i.e. to become a recognized culture of growth for all in that community and a resource within its geographic region for successful aging). To date, sixteen senior living communities have become designated and are leading the way for a major paradigm shift in how we see and experience aging in such communities. (See appendix for listing).

A strategic alliance with Sodexo Senior Living in early 2013 was a major step in the advancement of the Masterpiece Living approach to authentic health and successful aging. Sodexo is a quality-of-life services partner of over six hundred senior-living communities throughout the United States, specializing in building services, dining and nutrition, health and wellness, and strategic planning. In a total of more than 1,500 locations in the United States, Sodexo works to improve the quality of life for the customers, clients, and communities served. In schools and universities, in healthcare facilities and senior communities, in corporations and government sites, Sodexo's commitment to making every day a better day is constant. This partnership extended the potential reach of Masterpiece Living even beyond older adults. Such visionary leadership in a health-related industry is a positive sign that we can indeed not only manage health and aging but also can make it work for us as a nation.

We must continue to reach out to where most older adults actually live—in their homes, in towns and cities—and where they congregate: in senior centers (that name *will* change!), clubs, organizations, volunteer groups, and other places where they search for lives with meaning. The approach that is working so well for the thousands within our growing network can work for these people, and, I'm certain, for you. We will find ways to reach out to you, like the Sun Health outreach initiative in Phoenix, or citywide initiatives like that being considered in Puyallup, Washington and Ponca City, Oklahoma, our recent partnership with The

First Baptist Church of Jacksonville, Florida, or programs like that of the Four Pointes Center for Successful Aging. Creative partnerships such as these will enable you to find out what is possible and how to achieve it, to have the tools and resources to help you evaluate and modify your lifestyle, can find coaching support and environments that will make aging successfully a natural occurrence. We are committed to that goal.

The growing number of inspiring stories like the ones you have read about in this book, and like the ones in the national data bank we are accumulating, will provide us powerful tools to influence those still burdened with unenlightened views of aging. As the evidence grows stronger and stronger, it will become clear that public policy must reflect this new view of aging. Our vision of a country—indeed, a world—where *all* can continue to grow and be engaged, vital, valued, and needed is becoming clearer. After two and a half centuries of blurring misinterpretation, we are restoring not only hope but also respect and appreciation for a vast pool of untapped potential.

When we began the journey of growing a network, Masterpiece Living was a solid product. However, we knew we were not done refining it. We, in fact, will never be done. We will continue to learn more about the complex and magnificent process of aging and will incorporate this new knowledge into all we do. Aging as growing is an idea whose time has come, and the seismic nature of what it can mean for individuals and societies is palpable. Our journey from a taxicab ride with Jonas Salk to a validated approach to successful aging may have been a long one, but we are certain it has not been wasted. We look forward to the road ahead, for we know we are not alone. We know that we are traveling in the company of thousands of older adults who are committed to realizing their full potential no matter what life has in store for them. We're traveling with aging-services professionals who are not satisfied to just offer care, comfort, and security; with senior-living organizations, such as those noted in the appendix of this book, who are leading the way in the transformation of retirement communities; with passionate entrepreneurs such as Colin Milner of the International Council on Active Aging, Jack York of It's Never 2 Late, Kay Van Norman of Brilliant Aging, Maestro David Dworkin of Conductorcise, and Beth Sanders of LifeBio, all of whom, recognizing what is necessary to age in a better way, have developed resources to assist older adults in doing just that; and we're traveling with all who wish for a world where they will grow old with relevance. No, we're not traveling alone but in an ever-growing convoy more appropriately called a movement.

THE TIME OF OUR LIVES ... REALLY

I would rather be ashes than dust!
I would rather that my spark should burn out in a
brilliant blaze than it should be stifled by dry rot.
I would rather be a superb meteor, every atom of me in
magnificent glow, than a sleepy and permanent planet.
The proper function of man is to live, not to exist.

—JACK LONDON

These stirring words were written by the great author and adventurer, Jack London. Leave it to Jack to say it much better than I did with my leaf analogy. And what about you? How do you want to live? What do you want the rest of your life to be?

I hope your journey with me through this book has been enlightening, but more importantly, empowering. Jack London's credo, my hope, your wish for the rest of your life—all these *are* possible. As Yoda counsels, "Do or do not. There is no try." It is indeed only a matter of decision. The rest will happen. You will not fail. I'm sure of it. I've seen it in the thousands of older adults who honored me by allowing me to play a small part in their lives. How can I be so certain?

I'm certain because we know now that so much more is possible. We can indeed continue to grow physically, intellectually, socially, and spiritually throughout our lifespan. And these possibilities are dependent mostly on our lifestyle rather than our genes or luck or fate; it is our *choices* that are the major determinants of the quality—and for many, the quantity—of our lives.

I'm certain because we have a standard with which to evaluate the avalanche of miracle cures, health and fitness claims, medical information and advice, and diet and weight-loss information that can indeed leave us overwhelmed. We have a set of basic guidelines to act as a solid base to maneuver through the growing volume of health and aging advice. Those guidelines, of course, are the core set of needs firmly rooted in our DNA over the eons when our human ancestors were struggling to survive and to flourish. Needs which, I believe, are distinctly human—authentically human. The need to move, to be socially connected, to have a strong purpose, to be close to the natural world, and to eat foods provided by the earth and not factories. Whatever lifestyle choices you are considering, ask yourself if those choices are consistent with this standard, this core set of authentic principles for living and aging well. If yes, you're on course. If not, then you should seriously consider the value of those choices.

I'm certain you will not fail because if you use the principles of kaizen, of small, achievable steps that you establish and modify along the way, you cannot fail. If you do nothing, you won't fail, but you will most likely not age successfully either. If you do something, however modest, on a timetable determined by your progress, you will improve. You will be healthier. You will be aging in a better way. In fact, the commitment itself to live a lifestyle of continuous growth should *be* the goal, for successful aging will accompany that commitment.

I'm certain you will become healthier and age in a better way because the Ten Tips are a solid foundation for success. They are authentic, addressing the core needs we have as a species. They are holistic, not only because they address the full range of our health and aging needs but because they acknowledge the *absolute necessity* to address all. The Ten Tips are easy, for they are completely customizable to help you grow in all dimensions of your life.

You will not fail because no longer will stress be an invisible, silent destroyer of all that can be good in our lives, no longer the invasive killer of our bodies, our brains, and our souls. The Big Uneasy has been outed in this book and in the new research on aging, fully exposed as a by-product of an environment we were never designed to live in and empowered by our own thoughts and lack of mindfulness. So, now that it's exposed, it's vulnerable to our attention and to our desire to live lives free from fear, anxiety, and the illness that these bring. Stress need not be the constant, unwanted companion in our lives. We can be the masters of our internal selves and choose to be serene and fully present to all the beauty that is around us, seeing each moment as the gift it is and reaping the huge health rewards that are associated with that freedom from chronic stress.

Yes, you are now a warrior for a healthier life. You will not fail in your efforts to become authentically healthy. You will age in a better way—successfully, now that you know the stakes of inaction, now that you have guidelines, now that you know how to win over stress, now that you know you must pay attention to the physical, intellectual, social, and spiritual parts of you. You will not fail. I'm sure of it.

Facing a challenge doesn't mean you've failed

Let's get something straight before we end our journey together and begin a new one. Just because you encounter conditions commonly seen as one ages, from arthritis to cancer to heart disease, *does not mean you've failed.* Let me say it another way. Getting cancer, or heart disease, or even cognitive impairment doesn't mean it's your fault. It just means you must *deal with it* if you are to age successfully. Maybe it was something you did that made you more susceptible, maybe it wasn't. But this is a fork in the road for you. Your life's long path has crossed one of the many threats to aging well, and if you're going to stay on your current path to high performance and successful aging, then you must accept its presence and manage it to maximize the quality of your life. No beating the breast. No "Oh, woe is me" or "Why me?" or "I should have prevented this." There are, in fact, three kinds of prevention. Primary prevention is all about preventing new cases of a disease or condition. Secondary prevention is about identifying disease and conditions early in order to limit the spread or impact of the disease. And tertiary prevention is about minimizing the negative effects of the condition by treating symptoms and complications.

Let's say you have a family history of heart disease but no evidence that you have it. You don't smoke, you keep fit and lean, and you get your lipids and blood pressure checked regularly. This is *primary* prevention. You get some chest pain. You undergo an exercise-tolerance test and perhaps a cardiac catheterization and some X-ray studies. They find some early atherosclerotic heart disease. They insert a stint and prescribe some medication, exercise, and diet. This is *secondary* prevention. You have a heart attack and some of your heart muscle dies and you begin to get short of breath. They take care of the fluid backup, give you oxygen, and insert a pacemaker and prescribe cardiac rehabilitation exercises. This is *tertiary* prevention.

So, I'll say it once again, for it is critically important to understand. Aging successfully is about avoiding or preventing occurrence of a disease or condition whenever possible, *or* identifying it early to prevent it from taking hold, *or*, if it does become established, limiting its negative effects. Beating yourself up about the fact that you do have the condition is useless, destructive garbage.

Even death is not failing. We're all going to die. There is nothing we can do that will change that. We can and should prescribe advance directives to ensure our wishes are respected. But how we die—now there is something we can do something about. When? Maybe we can have an effect. But how? That *is* something we have a say in. For most of us, what our last days, weeks, even years are like can definitely be influenced by our actions, our attitude, our lifestyle. As my leaf metaphor and the title of this book suggest, we can do something about whether we end our days in a long, drawn-out, expensive, physically and emotionally painful and degrading process, or whether we minimize the time we are impaired. How we live our lives now has a very high probability of influencing the overall quality of our final curtain call.

The Movement calls

And as you move toward authentic health and successful aging, you will be part of a changing world: a world awakening to the possibility that aging is a privilege; that the current story of aging is one-dimensional, negatively deterministic, and wrong; that an aging population offers not only problems but solutions to the challenges of a quickly evolving society.

Live Long, Die Short is a call to action. Each of us, the organizations we belong to, the towns and cities we live in, and the societies that we have built—none of us can ignore the fact that we are aging, that usual aging isn't good enough anymore, and that much more is now possible. This not only calls for us to acknowledge this new reality but also presents us with a moral imperative: We must fundamentally shift the paradigm that marginalizes our older adults, that sees older adults as "accounts payable," and that takes a paternalistic view of the old. This paradigm shift will, as they say, "rock our world," as well it should. We must advocate for a public policy that acknowledges the potential of older adults not only to grow but also to become the solutions to many of our seemingly unsolvable challenges.

Together we *must* act. For each of us. For our grandchildren. For our community. For our world. For a world where aging is a revered part of our life's journey. And now that we know it's possible, don't we all have a responsibility to bring it to reality? We in Masterpiece Living are committed to bringing a culture of growth and successful aging not only to retirement communities but also to all living in their homes in towns and cities throughout this country and beyond. When you succeed in your life, when others succeed, when organizations succeed, when towns and cities succeed, it becomes a movement, paving the way for changes in public policy that will make aging a journey of wonder, adventure, and continued growth, policy that will make aging as colorful as New England fall leaves, where everyone has the possibility of living long and dying short.

MASTERPIECE LIVING PARTNERS

SYSTEM	HEADQUARTERS
ABHOW	Pleasanton, CA
Ascension Health/Via Christi	St. Louis, MO
be.group	Glendale, CA
Celebration Village	Johns Creek, GA
Christian Living Communities	Greenwood Village, CO
Community Wellness Partners	New Hartford, NY
Episcopal Communities & Services	Pasadena, CA
Hallman Retirement Neighborhoods	Pottstown, PA
Lifespace Communities, Inc.	Des Moines, IA
Lutheran Senior Services	St. Louis, MO
Masonic Homes of CA	Union City, CA
Ohio Presbyterian Retirement Services	Cincinnati, OH
Presbyterian SeniorCare	Verona, PA
Presbyterian Senior Living	Dillsburg, PA
Sage Senior Living	Philadelphia, PA
Senior Villages	Brighton, MI
Solvere Senior Living	Princeton, NJ
SQLC	Dallas, TX
Sun Health	Phoenix, AZ

MASTERPIECE LIVING COMMUNITY PARTNERS

Redstone Village	Huntsville, AL
Grandview Terrace	Sun City West, AZ
La Loma Village	Litchfield Park, AZ

Sun Health Senior Living. . . . . .Surprise, AZ

The Colonnade . . . . .Surprise, AZ

The Terraces of Phoenix . . . . .Phoenix, AZ

Acacia Creek . . . . .Union City, CA

Casa de la Vista. . . . . .Redlands, CA

Fern Lodge. . . . . .Redlands, CA

Grand Lake Gardens . . . . .Oakland, CA

Masonic Homes of Union City. . . . . .Union City, CA

MonteCedro . . . . .Pasadena, CA

Piedmont Gardens .Oakland, CA

Plymouth Village . . . . .Redlands, CA

Rosewood Senior Living . . . . .Bakersfield, CA

The Terraces at Los Altos. . . . . .Los Altos, CA

The Terraces at Los Gatos . . . . .Los Gatos, CA

The Terraces at San Joaquin Gardens. . . . . .Fresno, CA

Clermont Park. . . . . .Denver, CO

Holly Creek Retirement Community . . . . .Centennial, CO

Someren Glen . . . . .Centennial, CO

Elim Park. . . . . .Cheshire, CT

Westminster Village in Dover. . . . . .Dover, DE

Abbey Delray. . . . . .Delray Beach, FL

Abbey Delray South . . . . .Delray Beach, FL

First Baptist Church . . . . .Jacksonville, FL

Harbour's Edge . . . . .Delray Beach, FL

The Waterford . . . . .Juno Beach, FL

Village on the Green. . . . . .Longwood, FL

Celebration Village - Acworth . . . . .Acworth, GA

Celebration Village - Forsyth . . . . .Forsyth, GA

Deerfield Retirement Community . . . . . . .Urbandale, IA

Beacon Hill . . . . .Lombard, IL

Meridian Village . . . . .Glen Carbon, IL

Oak Trace. . . . . .Downers Grove , IL

The Birches . . . . .Clarendon Hills, IL

The Barrington at Carmel . . . . .Carmel, IN

Catholic Care Center . . . . .Bel Aire, KS

Claridge Court . . . . .Prairie Village, KS

Glen Meadows. . . . . .Glen Arm, MD

Four Pointes Center for Successful Aging. .Grand Haven, MI

StoryPoint at Rockford. . . . . .Rockford, MI

Friendship Village of Bloomington . . . . . .Bloomington, MN

Breeze Park . . . . .St. Charles, MO

Heisinger Bluffs. . . . . .Jefferson City, MO

Salemtowne . . . . .Winston-Salem, NC

Grand Lodge at the Preserve. . . . . .Lincoln, NE

Arbor Glen. . . . . .Bridgewater, NJ

Homestead at Hamilton. . . . . .Hamilton, NJ

Las Ventanas . . . . .Summerlin, NV

Peconic Landing . . . . .Greenport, NY

Presbyterian Home .New Hartford, NY

Presbyterian Residential Community . . . . .New Hartford, NY

Preswick Glen . . . . .New Hartford, NY

The Brielle at Seaview. . . . . .Staten Island, NY

The Meadows. . . . . .New Hartford, NY

Independence Village at Avon Park . . . . . . .Avon Park, OH

Llanfair. . . . . .Cincinnati, OH

Cathedral Village . . . . .Philadelphia, PA

Daylesford Crossing . . . . .Paoli, PA

Friendship Village of South Hills . . . . .Upper St. Clair, PA

Green Ridge Valley. .Newville, PA

Kirkland Village . . . . .Bethlehem, PA

Kyffin Grove. . . . . .North Wales, PA

Longwood at Oakmont . . . . .Verona, PA

Plush Mills. . . . . .Wallingford, PA

Presbyterian Home at Williamsport . . . . . .Williamsport, PA

Presbyterian Village at Hollidaysburg . . . . .Hollidaysburg, PA

Quincy Village. . . . . .Waynesboro, PA

Santoga Ridge Community . . . . .Pottstown, PA

St. Andrew's Village .Indiana, PA

The Easton Home . . . . .Easton, PA

The Long Community at Highland . . . . . . .Lancaster, PA

Ware Presbyterian Village . . . . .Oxford, PA

Wesley House at Quincy Village. . . . . .Waynesboro, PA

Westminster Village-Allentown . . . . .Allentown, PA

Westminster Woods at Huntingdon . . . . . .Huntingdon, PA

Windy Hill Village .Philipsburg, PA

Woodland Retirement Community. . . . . . .Orbisonia, PA

The Woodlands at Furman . . . . .Greenville, SC

Edgemere. . . . . .Dallas, TX

Lutheran Sunset . . . . .Clifton, TX

Mirador . . . . .Corpus Christi, TX

Querencia at Barton Creek . . . . .Austin, TX

The Buckingham. . . . . .Houston, TX

The Stayton at Museum Way. . . . . .Fort Worth, TX

Judson Park . . . . .Des Moines, WA

Eastcastle Place . . . . .Milwaukee, WI

CERTIFIED CENTERS FOR SUCCESSFUL AGING

Acacia Creek . . . . .Union City, CA

Clermont Park. . . . . .Denver, CO

Edgemere. . . . . .Dallas, TX

Holly Creek . . . . .Greenwood Village, CO

Judson Park . . . . .Des Moines, WA

Las Ventanas . . . . .Las Vegas, NV

Plymouth Village . . . . .Redlands, CA

Presbyterian Village at Hollidaysburg . . . . .Hollidaysburg, PA

Querencia at Barton Creek . . . . .Austin, TX

Quincy Village. . . . . .Waynesboro, PA

Rosewood . . . . .Bakersfield, CA

Someren Glen . . . . .Centennial, CO

The Buckingham . . . . .Houston, TX

The Stayton at Museum Way. . . . . .Ft. Worth, TX

The Terraces at San Joaquin Gardens. . . . . .Fresno, CA

The Terraces of Phoenix . . . . .Phoenix, AZ

NOTES

Introduction

1. John Wallace Rowe and Robert L. Kahn, *Successful Aging* (New York: Dell, 1998), 38.

Part I Introduction

1. Merriam-Webster online, s.v. "authentic," http://www.merriam-webster.com/dictionary/authentic.

Chapter 1

1. René Dubois, introduction to Norman Cousins, *Anatomy of an Illness* (New York: Bantam Books, 1981).

2. Jon Kabat-Zinn, address to Cape Cod Community College, August 2, 2012.

3. BrainyQuote, http://www.brainyquote.com/quotes/quotes/j/joandving224859.html.

4. Jared Diamond, *The World Until Yesterday* (New York: Viking Penguin, 2012.)

5. Robert Wright, *The Moral Animal* (New York: Vintage, 1994).

6. David Brody, *The Other Side of Eden* (New York: Faber & Faber, 2001).

7. Marjorie Shostak, *Nisa: The Life and Words of a !Kung Woman* (Cambridge, MA: Harvard University Press, 2001).

8. Simone de Beauvoir, *The Coming of Age* (New York: W. W. Norton, 1970).

9. PBS.org, *American Experience: The Richest Man in the World: Andrew Carnegie,* http://www.pbs.org/wgbh/amex/carnegie/sfeature/mf_steelworker.html.

10. Liam J. Donaldson and Raymond J. Donaldson, *Esssential Public Health* (London: Radcliffe, 2005), 105.

11. Wright, *Moral Animal.*

12. Paola Scommegna, "U.S. Growing Bigger, Older, and More Diverse," April 2004, http://www.prb.org/Articles/2004/USGrowingBiggerOlderandMoreDiverse.aspx.

13. Ken Dychtwald, *Age Wave* (New York: Bantam, 1990).

14. Ken Dychtwald, *Age Power* (New York: Jeremy P. Tarcher / Putnam, 1999), front cover.

15. Dychtwald, *Age Power.*

Chapter 2

1. Robert Butler, *Why Survive? Being Old in America* (Baltimore: Johns Hopkins University Press, 1975).

2. James Freis, keynote address to the Institute of Medicine, National Academy of Sciences, Washington, DC, October 1982.

3. Centers for Disease Control and Prevention, "Death and Mortality," http://www.cdc.gov/nchs/fastats/deaths.htm.

4. Dan Buettner, "The Secrets of Longevity," *National Geographic,* November 2005; Buettner, *The Blue Zones* (Washington, DC: The National Geographic Society, 2008).

5. Buettner, *Blue Zones.*

Chapter 3

1. Thomas Perls and Paola Sebastiani, "The Genetics of Extreme Longevity: Lessons from the New England Centenarian Study," *Frontiers in Genetics* 3, article 277, November 2012.

2. James Prochaska and Carlo DiClemente, *The Transtheoretical Approach: Crossing the Traditional Boundaries of Therapy* (Melbourne, Florida: Krieger Publishing Company, 1994).

3. Robert Maurer, *One Small Step Can Change Your Life: The Kaizen Way* (New York: Workman, 2004).

4. Maurer, *One Small Step.*

5. Ian Robertson, *Mind Sculpture: Unlocking Your Brain's Untapped Potential* (New York: Fromm International Publishing Corporation, 2001).

6. Maurer, *One Small Step.*

Tip 1

1. Joan Vernikos, *The G-Connection* (Lincoln, NE: iUniverse, 2004), 57.

2. Y. Nigam, J. Knight, and A. Jones, "Effects of Bedrest 3: Musculoskeletal and Immune Systems, Skin and Self-perception," *Nursing Times* 105: 18–22, 2009.

3. D.L. Waters, R.N. Baumgartner, and P.J. Garry, "Sarcopenia: Current Perspectives," *The Journal of Nutrition, Health & Aging* 4 (3): 133-139, 2000.

4. Frank W. Booth and Manu V. Chakravarthy, "Cost and Consequences of Sedentary Living: New Battleground For an Old Enemy," President's Council on Physical Fitness and Sports's *Research Digest,* series 3, no. 16, March 2002.

5. Ellen Langer, *Counterclockwise: Mindful Health and the Power of Possibility* (New York: Ballantine Books, 2009).

6. Anna S. Mueller, et al, "Sizing up Peers: Adolescent Girls' Weight Control and Social Comparison in the School Context," *Journal of Health and Social Behavior* 51 (1): 64–78, 2010.

7. Nicholas A. Christakis and James H. Fowler, "The Spread of Obesity in a Large Social Network over 32 Years," *New England Journal of Medicine* 357: 370–379, July 26, 2007.

8.   Richard Louv, *Last Child in the Woods: Saving Our Children from Nature Deficit Disorder* (Chapel Hill, NC: Algonquin Books, 2008).

Tip 2

1.   John R. Pleis, Jacqueline W. Lucas, Brian W. Ward, *Summary Health Statistics for U.S. Adults: National Health Interview Survey*, Series Reports from the National Health Interview Survey #10, Centers for Disease Control and Prevention, p. 11, http://www.cdc.gov/nchs/data/series/sr_10/sr10_242.pdf.

2.   Pleis et al., *Summary Health Statistics.*

3.   Frank W. Booth, Scott E. Gordon, Christian J. Carlson, and Marc T. Hamilton, "Waging War on Modern Chronic Diseases: Primary Prevention Through Exercise Biology," *Journal of Applied Physiology* 88, 774–787, 2000, http://jap.physiology.org/content/88/2/774.full.pdf.

4.   Frank W. Booth and Manu V. Chakravarthy, "Cost and Consequences of Sedentary Living: New Battleground For an Old Enemy," President's Council on Physical Fitness and Sports's *Research Digest,* series 3, no. 16, March 2002.

5.   Adapted from "Chronic Diseases Caused or Enhanced by Three Risk Factors: Smoking, Obesity, and Sedentary Lifestyle" in "Expanding Your Model: Optimizing Referrals and Introducing Disease Management" by Linda K. Hall, in William E. Kraus and Steven J. Keteyian, eds., *Cardiac Rehabilitation* (Totowa, NJ: Humana Press, 2007), 258.

6.   Booth and Chakravarthy, "Cost and Consequences," 4.

7.   Russell R. Pate, Michael Platt, Steven N. Blair, et al., "Physical Activity and Public Health—A Recommendation from the Centers for Disease Control and Prevention and the American College of Sports Medicine," *Journal of the American Medical Association* 273 (5): 402–407, February 1995.

8.   J. Michael McGinnis and William H. Foege, "Actual Causes of Death in the United States," *Journal of the American Medical Association* 270 (18): 2207–2212, November 1993.

9.   REF Power 9® Reverse Engineering Longevity posted on April 9, 2014 by Dan Buettner.

10.   The study published in *Annals of Internal Medicine* was led by Biswas, research student at Toronto Rehab, UHN and the Institute of Health Policy, Management and Evaluation, University of Toronto, and the senior author is Dr. Alter.

Tip 3

1.   Alvaro Fernandez and Elkhonon Goldberg, *The SharpBrains Guide to Brain Fitness* (San Francisco: SharpBrains, 2009).

2.   MedicineNet.com, definition of "neuroplasticity," http://www.medterms.com/script/main/art.asp?articlekey=40362.

3. Jill Bolte Taylor, *My Stroke of Insight* (New York: Penguin, 2006).

4. Eileen Luders, Arthur W. Toga, Natasha Lepore, and Christian Gaser, "The Underlying Anatomical Correlates of Long-term Meditation: Larger Hippocampal and Frontal Volumes of Gray Matter," *Neuroimage* 45, (3): 672–678, April 15, 2009.

5. David Snowdon, *Aging with Grace* (New York: Bantam, 2001).

6. Fiona Matthews, Carol Brayne, et al., "A Two Decade Comparison of Prevalence of Dementia in Individuals Aged 65 Years and Older from Three Geographical Areas in England: Results of the Cognitive Function and Ageing Study 1 & 2," *The Lancet* (July 17, 2013), doi:10.1016/S0140-6736(13)61570-6; Kaare Christensen et al., "Physical and Cognitive Functioning of People Older Than 90 Years: A Comparison of Two Danish Cohorts Born 10 Years Apart," *The Lancet* (July 11, 2013), doi: 10.1016/S0140-6736(13)60777-1.

7. Robert Winningham, *Train Your Brain* (Amityville, NY: Baywood Publishing Company, 2010).

8. Guy McKhann and Marilyn Albert, *Keep Your Brain Young* (Hoboken, NJ: Wiley, 2002).

9. Sandra Bond Chapman, *Make Your Brain Smarter* (New York: Free Press, 2013).

10. PBS / Santa Fe Productions, *The Distracted Mind, with Dr. Adam Gazzaley,* 2013.

11. Youfa Wang, M. A. Beydoun, and H. A. Beydoun, "Obesity and Central Obesity as Risk Factors for Incident Dementia and Its Subtypes," *Obesity Reviews,* 9 (3): 204–218, May 2008.

12. Chapman, *Make Your Brain Smarter.*

Tip 4

1. Robert Wright, *The Moral Animal* (New York: Vintage, 1994).

2. Paul MacLean, *The Triune Brain in Evolution* (New York: Plenum Press, 1990).

3. Thomas Lewis, Fari Amini, and Richard Lannon, *A General Theory of Love* (New York: Random House, 2000).

4. Robert Kahn and Toni Antonucci, "Convoys Over the Life Course: Attachment, Roles, and Social Support," *Life-Span Development and Behavior,* 3: 253–286, June 1980.

5. Nicholas Baker, Florian Wolschin, and Gro Amdam, "Age-Related Learning Deficits Can Be Reversible in Honeybees *Apis mellifera*," *Experimental Gerontology,* 47 (10): 764–772, October 2012.

6. Giacomo Rizzolatti and Laila Craighero, "The Mirror-Neuron System," *Annual Review of Neuroscience,* 27: 169–192, July 2004.

7.   Robert Putnam, *Bowling Alone* (New York: Simon & Schuster, 2000).

8.   L. F. Glass and T. Berkman, "Social Integration, Social Networks, Social Support and Health," *Social Epidemiology* (New York: Oxford University Press, 2000).

9.   Putnam, *Bowling Alone.*

10. William B. Malarkey, Ronald Glaser, Janice K. Kiecolt-Glaser, and Phillip T. Marucha, "Behavior: The Endocrine-Immune Interface and Health Outcomes," *Advances in Psychosomatic Medicine,* 22: 104–115, 2001.

11. Seligman, Martin, "Boomer Blues" *Psychology Today,* October 1988.

12. Julianne Holt-Lunstad, Timothy Smith, and J. Bradley Layton, "Social Relationships and Mortality Risk: A Meta-Analytic Review," *PLOS Medicine* 7, July 2010.

13. Kevin Hogan and Ron Stubbs, *Can't Get Through: 8 Barriers to Communication* (Gretna, LA: Pelican Publishing Company, 2003).

14. Miller McPherson, Matthew Brashears, and Lynn Smith-Lovin, "Social Isolation in America: Changes in Core Discussion Networks over Two Decades," *American Sociological Review,* 71: 353–375, June 2006.

15. Sherry Turkle, *Alone Together: Why We Expect More From Technology and Less From Each Other* (New York: Basic Books, 2011).

Tip 5

1.   J. Michael McGinnis and William H. Foege, "Actual Causes of Death in the United States," *Journal of the American Medical Association* 270 (18): 2207–2212, November 1993.

2.   Sun Tzu, *The Art of War,* translated by Samuel B. Griffith (Oxford: Clarendon Press, 1963).

3.   Sarah French, Michael Rosenberg, and Matthew Knuiman, "The Clustering of Health Risk Behaviours in a Western Adult Population," *Health Promotion Journal of Australia* 3 (19): 203–209, December 2008.

4.   Robert M. Sapolsky, foreword to Bruce McEwen, *The End of Stress As We Know It* (Atlanta, GA: Joseph Henry Press, 2002).

5.   Bruce McEwen, *The End of Stress As We Know It* (Atlanta, GA: Joseph Henry Press, 2002).

6.   McEwen, *End of Stress.*

7.   Sheldon Cohen, Denise Janicki-Deverts, and Gregory Miller, "Psychological Stress and Disease," *Journal of the American Medical Association* 298 (14): 1687–1689, October 2007.

8.   Roland Sturm, *The Health Risks of Obesity: Worse Than Smoking, Drinking, or Poverty,* RAND Health research brief, 2002, http://www.rand.org/pubs/research_briefs/RB4549.html.

9. Solomon H. Katz, *Encyclopedia of Food and Culture* (Farmington Hills, MI: Gale, 2003).

10. United States Department of Agriculture, http://www.choosemyplate.gov.

Tip 6

1. Bradley J. Willcox, D. Craig Willcox, and Makoto Suzuki, *The Okinawa Program* (New York: Three Rivers Press, 2001).

2. Ellen J. Langer, *Counterclockwise* (New York: Ballantine, 2009).

Tip 7

1. Viktor Frankl, *The Doctor and the Soul* (New York: Vintage, 1986).

2. Harold G. Koenig, Michael E. McCullough, and David Larson, *Handbook of Religion and Health* (Oxford: Oxford University Press, 2001).

3. Thomas Moore, *Care of the Soul* (New York: HarperCollins, 1992).

4. Lars Tornstam, *Gerotranscendence* (New York: Springer, 2005).

5. Harry Moody, *The Five Stages of the Soul* (New York: Anchor, 1997).

6. Eckhart Tolle, *The Power of Now* (New World Library / Namaste Publishing, 1999).

7. Robert Sapolsky, *Why Zebras Don't Get Ulcers* (New York: Holt, 1994).

8. Tolle, *Power of Now.*

9. Moore, *Care of the Soul.*

10. Eileen Luders, Arthur W. Toga, Natasha Lepore, and Christian Gaser, "The Underlying Anatomical Correlates of Long-term Meditation: Larger Hippocampal and Frontal Volumes of Gray Matter," *Neuroimage* 45 (3): 672–678, April 15, 2009.

11. McEwen, *End of Stress.*

12. Eileen Luders, Nicolas Cherbuin, Florian Kurth. Forever Young(er): potential age-defying effects of long-term meditation on gray matter atrophy. *Frontiers in Psychology*, 2015; 5 DOI: 10.3389/fpsyg.2014.01551)

13. McEwen, *End of Stress.*

Tip 8

1. Erik Erikson, *Childhood and Society* (New York: Norton, 1950).

2. Erik Erikson, Joan Erikson, and Helen Kivnick, *Vital Involvement in Old Age* (New York: Norton, 1986).

3. Eden Alternative website, "Our Ten Principles," accessed July 30, 2013, http://www.edenalt.org/our-10-principles.

4. Robert Grimm Jr., Kimberly Spring, and Nathan Dietz, *The Health Benefits of Volunteering: A Review of Recent Research* (Washington, DC: Corporation for National and Community Service, Office of Research and Policy Development y, 2007).

5. "The Value of Volunteering," Masterpiece Living, accessed August 14, 2013, http://www.mymasterpieceliving.com/index.cfm?fuseaction=content.Successful_Aging_Data_Revelations.

6. Steven Cole, et al., "A Functional Genomic Perspective on Human Well-Being," *Proceedings of the National Academy of Sciences* 110 (33): 13684–13689, published ahead of print, July 29, 2013.

7. Richard Leider, *The Power of Purpose* (San Francisco: Berrett-Koehler, 2004).

8. Mark Gerzon, *Coming Into Our Own* (New York: Delacorte, 1992).

Tip 9

1. "Humana and KaBoom! Kick Off 2nd Annual Multigenerational Playground Builds," Humana press release, September 20, 2012, http://press.humana.com/press-release/current-releases/humana-and-kaboom-kick-2nd-annual-multigenerational-playground-builds.

2. Joseph Tierney, Jean Baldwin Grossman, and Nancy Resch, *Making a Difference: An Impact Study of Big Brothers Big Sisters* (Philadelphia, PA: Public/Private Ventures, 2000).

3. Elza Maria de Souza, "Intergenerational Integration, Social Capital and Health: A Theoretical Framework and Results from a Qualitative Study," *Ciencia & Saluda Coletiva* 16 (3): 1733–1744, March 2011.

4. Janice Lloyd, "Temple University Achieves Intergenerational Excellence," *USA Today*, October 24, 2011.

Tip 10

1. Hans Selye, *The Stress of Life* (New York: McGraw-Hill, 1978).

2. Norman Cousins, *Anatomy of an Illness* (New York: Norton, 1979).

3. Thomas Perls and Paola Sebastiani, "The Genetics of Extreme Longevity: Lessons from the New England Centenarian Study," *Frontiers in Genetics* 3, article 277, November 2012.

4. Jeanie Lerche Davis, "Why Do We Laugh," WebMD feature, http://men.webmd.com/features/why-do-we-laugh.

5. L. Berk, D. Felten, S. Tan, B. Bittman, and J. Westengard, "Modulation of Neuroimmune Parameters During the Eustress of Humor-associated Mirthful Laughter," *Alternative Therapies in Health and Medicine* 7: 62–72, 74–6. 2001.

6. R. I. M. Dunbar et al., "Social Laughter Correlated with an Elevated Pain Threshold," *Proceedings of the Royal Society B: Biological Sciences,* 279 (1731): 1161–1167, March 2012.

7. American Physiological Society, "Laughter Remains Good Medicine," *Science Daily,* April 17, 2009.

8. Dalai Lama, *My Spiritual Journey* (New York: HarperCollins, 2011).

9. Langer, *Counterclockwise.*

Chapter 16

1. Ken Dychtwald, *Age Power* (New York: Jeremy P. Tarcher/Putnam, 1999).
2. Bill Thomas, "Eldertopia," AARP International's *The Journal,* Summer 2011.
3. Zalman Schachter-Shalomi, *From Age-ing to Sage-ing* (New York: Warner Books, 1995).
4. David Gutman, *Reclaimed Powers* (New York: Basic Books, 1987).
5. John R. Beard, Simon Biggs, David E. Bloom, Linda P. Fried, Paul Hogan, Alexandre Kalache, and S. Jay Olshansky, eds., *Global Population Ageing: Peril or Promise* (Geneva: World Economic Forum, 2011).
6. Malcolm Gladwell, *The Tipping Point* (New York: Little Brown, 2000).
7. Katie Sloan, address to the Masterpiece Living Lyceum, February 2011.

Chapter 17

1. National Center for Chronic Disease Prevention & Health Promotion, "The Power of Prevention: Chronic Disease . . . the Public Health Challenge of the 21st Century," Washington, DC: Centers for Disease Control and Prevention, 2009).
2. *Code of Federal Regulations,* Quality of Life, title 42, sec. 483.15.
3. Conclusions of the 2011 Strategy Session, International Council on Active Aging, Bethesda, MD.
4. J. A. Stevens, P. S. Corso, E. A. Finkelstein, T. R. Miller, "The Costs of Fatal and Nonfatal Falls Among Older Adults," *Injury Prevention* 12 (5): 290–295, 2006.
5. F. Englander, T. J. Hodson, and R. A. Terregrossa, "Economic Dimensions of Slip and Fall Injuries," *Journal of Forensic Science* 41 (5): 733–746, 1996. M.C. Hombrook, V.J. Stevens, D.J. Wingfield, et al., "Preventing Falls Among Community-Dwelling Older Persons: Results from a Randomized Trial," *The Gerontologist* 34 (1): 16–23, 1994.
6. A. Shumway-Cook, M. A. Ciol, J. Hoffman, B. J. Dudgeon, K. Yorston, L. Chan, "Falls in the Medicare Population: Incidence, Associated Factors, and Impact on Health Care," *Physical Therapy* 89 (4): 1–9, 2009.
7. M. C. Robertson, A. J. Campbell, M. M. Gardner, et al., "Preventing Injuries in Older People by Preventing Falls: A Meta-analysis of Individual-Level Data," *Journal of American Geriatric Society* 50 (5): 905–11, May 2002.
8. Seth Godin, *Poke the Box* (Do You Zoom, Inc., 2011).
9. Marc Freedman, *The Big Shift* (New York: PublicAffairs, 2011).About the Author

INDEX

ABOUT THE AUTHOR

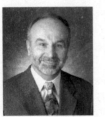 **DR. ROGER LANDRY** is a preventive-medicine physician who specializes in building environments that empower older adults to maximize their unique potential.

Trained at Tufts University School of Medicine and Harvard University School of Public Health, he is the president of Masterpiece Living, a group of multidiscipline specialists in aging who partner with communities to assist them in becoming destinations for continued growth.

Dr. Landry was a flight surgeon in the Air Force for over twenty-two years, keeping pilots and other aircrew healthy and performing at their best. One of his charges was world-famous test pilot Chuck Yeager. Dr. Landry retired as a highly decorated full colonel and chief flight surgeon at the Air Force Surgeon General's Office in Washington, DC, after duty on five continents and being medically involved in a number of significant world events, including Vietnam, the Chernobyl nuclear disaster, the Beirut bombing of the Marine barracks, the first seven shuttle launches, and the first manned balloon crossing of the Pacific.

For the last decade, Dr. Landry has focused his efforts on older adults as a lecturer, researcher, consultant, and author. He lives on Cape Cod.